D0210581

SECRETS
FROM THE
EATING LAB

SECRETS FROM THE EATING LAB

The Science of Weight Loss, the Myth of Willpower, and Why You Should Never Diet Again

....

TRACI MANN, PH.D.

HARPER WAVE

An Imprint of HarperCollinsPublishers

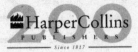

HarperCollins
PUBLISHERS
———— *Since 1817* ————

This book is written as a source of information only. The information contained in this book should by no means be considered a substitute for the advice of a qualified medical professional, who should always be consulted before beginning any new diet, exercise, or other health program. All efforts have been made to ensure the accuracy of the information contained in this book as of the date published. The author and the publisher expressly disclaim responsibility for any adverse effects arising from the use or application of the information contained herein.

HarperCollins books may be purchased for educational, business, or sales promotional use. For information, please e-mail the Special Markets Department at SPsales@harpercollins.com.

A hardcover edition of this book was published in 2015 by HarperWave, an imprint of HarperCollins Publishers.

FIRST HARPERWAVE PAPERBACK EDITION PUBLISHED 2017

Designed by William Ruoto

Library of Congress Cataloging-in-Publication Data

Mann, Traci.
  Secrets from the eating lab : the science of weight loss, the myth of willpower, and why you should never diet again / Traci Mann, PhD.
    pages cm
ISBN 978-0-06-232923-3 (hardback)
  1. Reducing diets—Social aspects. 2. Reducing diets—Psychological aspects.
3. Weight loss—Social aspects. 4. Weight loss—Psychological aspects. I. Title.
  RM222.2.M3257 2015
  613.2'5—dc23
                          2014049872
ISBN 978-0-06-232925-7 (pbk.)

  18 19 20 21   OV/RRD   10 9 8 7 6 5 4 3

In memory of my parents, Jacklyn Rosen Mann and Richard Mann, who died thin and too soon. In my fondest memories of them, they are healthy, happy, and fat.

And for my husband, Stephen Engel, for making this book possible.

CONTENTS

PART FOUR: YOUR WEIGHT IS REALLY NOT THE POINT

PREFACE

"You study self-control? You should study me.
I have great self-control."

—NOBODY, EVER

There is no sign on the door of the Health and Eating Lab at the University of Minnesota. That's my lab, and if I want to learn about people's eating habits, I can't let on that I am studying—or even noticing—what people are eating. It would make them self-conscious and stop them from eating the way they normally do. Instead, my students and I tell our research participants that we are studying other things entirely, such as their memory, or their moods, or how they communicate with their friends. But being the hospitable people we are, we just happen to offer them some snacks while we study them. They have no idea that it's what they do with those snacks that we're really studying.

For more than twenty years, I have been doing research on eating, both with sneaky studies in my eating lab on campus, and in that other eating lab known as "the real world," where I have studied dieters going about their normal daily routines, kids eating in school cafeterias, visitors to the annual feeding frenzy that is the Minnesota State Fair, and even astronauts on the International Space Station. Much to my surprise, I've learned that nearly everything I thought was true about eating was false, including the three pillars of the commercial diet industry: that diets work, that dieting is good for you, and that obesity is deadly. The truth is that diets do not work and may be bad for you, and obesity is not going to kill you. I also learned that despite what most people assume, a lack of self-control is not why people become fat and "harnessing" willpower is not the way to become thin.

Along the way I've also learned that many people have a vested interest in all of us believing those things are true. The obesity research community, in particular, is not delighted that my students and I dare to question their three sacred cows. I've had a well-known diet researcher publicly accuse my young graduate student of doing a disservice to the field by suggesting that diets don't lead to long-term weight loss. I've gotten such vitriolic reviews of manuscripts that journal editors have called me before sending the reviews to prepare me for what I was about to read. I've had journal editors unable to find scholars willing to provide reviews of my work (even negative reviews) out of fear of getting involved in a controversy. And I've received lots of hostile and decidedly nonscholarly feedback when I've spoken up about these things in the media. Some people discount my research by suggesting I must be a bitter fat person (as if fat people cannot be scientists). One online commenter said I was just looking for an excuse to continue stuffing myself "like a Thanksgiving turkey."

I'm not obese, but I am a science nerd, obsessed with research methods and data, and the results of my studies don't lie (or have anything to do with what I weigh). I can't ignore them and I do not want to, because my research points the way to living a healthy life without suggesting that dieting is the answer. And that way to living a healthier life is what I'll share with you in this book.

In Part I, I'll share the research that proves diets don't lead to long-term weight loss and explain why this is so. If you lost a lot of weight and then gained it back, it is not because you lack self-control. In fact, I suspect you used more self-control than the people who accuse you of not having any. But it doesn't matter either way. Self-control is not the problem, and harnessing it is not the solution.

In Part II, I will make the case that diets are neither harmless nor necessary for optimal health, and that most people simply should not go on restrictive diets. My argument is based on the scientific criteria doctors use when they decide whether to recommend treatments (such as drugs) to patients for other conditions: Does the treatment work? Is it safe? Does it have side effects? For some reason, people rarely ask these questions before urging everyone to diet, but my students and I asked them, and the answers are clear: no, not necessarily, yes.

I understand that we all have an image in our mind about what we want to weigh. The problem is that for many of us, that image is outside of our biologically set weight range. It is possible to maintain a weight outside that range—a small minority of dieters does—but to do so, you would have to make weight maintenance the central focus of your life, above all others, including your relationships with your family and friends, your work, and your emotional well-being. It would be a life of agonizing self-denial, and for what purpose?

Instead, I suggest we aim to live at the low end of our set weight range, which is our leanest livable weight. At that weight you can be happy and healthy, and you can maintain it without making it your life's work. In Part III we will look at twelve scientifically supported strategies for painlessly getting to that weight and staying there. These strategies don't involve calorie restriction or require willpower, because relying on willpower is foolhardy, and this is not a diet. Remember, I run an eating lab, not a dieting lab.

You won't find this set of strategies elsewhere, because most of them are based on the research conducted in my lab over the last two decades. Not only will the results of this research surprise you, but I suspect the methods we use in these studies will as well. A rule of thumb in my lab is that if there is a fun way to do a study and a boring way to do a study, we go with the fun way. And as we've learned, there's always a fun way. But rest assured, the methodology we use is rigorous. In fact, the goofier the methods, the more rigorous the study needs to be to get published in leading academic journals, as these studies are.

Finally, once you are effortlessly maintaining your leanest livable weight, in Part IV I'll urge you to forget about the numbers on the scale and get on with your life. That means you need to forget about other people's weight, too. Rebel against our weight-obsessed culture by fighting weight stigma, and shift the focus to your health and well-being instead of your weight. I'll introduce you to the reasonable—yet oddly unnoticed—notion that doing healthy things is healthy, whether or not they make you model-thin. Let's get started.

PART ONE

WHY DIETS FAIL YOU

· ·

CHAPTER 1

DIETS DON'T
WORK

Diets don't work. There. I said it. Maybe that's not what you wanted me to say, but I'm here to tell you the truth, according to science, without sugarcoating it. Like most simple-sounding scientific points, of course, it is more complicated than it seems. The reason for the complexity comes from the word "work." What you mean when you think of a diet "working" is not the same as what, say, the CEO of a diet company or an obesity researcher means.

I suspect that for you, a diet works if you lose a lot of weight and keep it off. If that's the case, I can tell you definitively: diets don't work. Diet company CEOs might define "works" a little differently: for them, a diet may work if people lose any weight at all for any length of time. And for obesity researchers, a diet might work if test subjects lose slightly more weight than people who are not dieting. CEOs and obesity researchers say diets work because people do lose weight—and more weight than non-dieters—during the early months of most diets. Since the 1940s, hundreds of studies have shown that dieters lose an average of five to fifteen pounds over the first four to six months on a diet.[1]

This seems to be the case no matter what type of diet you try, whether you go low calorie, low fat, or low carb, or whether you attempt whatever fad diet is currently popular. There are diets that require you to fast for hours or days at a time,[2] diets that require you to consume only liquids, diets that suggest you eat like a caveman, or even diets that restrict your food intake solely to grapefruit, cabbage soup, or Snickers bars.[3] There are also diets that promise to publicly humiliate you if you fail,[4] or jolt you with electric shocks whenever you attempt to eat certain foods. As recently as 2014, a doctor in the United States was sewing patches onto people's tongues to cause them stabbing pain whenever they ate.[5]

So when CEOs and obesity researchers say diets are effective, they are not technically lying, because diets do lead to weight loss in the short term. But there are two problems with saying these diets work: people don't lose enough weight, and they don't keep it off.

WHAT DOES IT MEAN FOR A DIET TO "WORK"?

Although it seems like a no-brainer to most dieters, it has been surprisingly difficult for the medical community to decide what constitutes a successful diet. Even deciding what counts as a "normal" weight is not as simple as you might think. The World Health Organization (WHO) currently classifies people's weights based on their body mass index, or BMI,[6] which is a measure of weight that takes height into account. The use of BMI is controversial because the formula for calculating it is not based on any understanding of how height and weight relate to each other, and because people who have high muscle mass tend to get categorized as overweight, despite having very little fat.[7] Nevertheless, according to the WHO,[8] the cutoff between what it calls normal weight[9] and overweight is a BMI of 25, and between overweight and obese is 30. Anything under 18.5 is considered underweight.

Originally, the goal of a diet was to achieve what was known as your "ideal weight." Starting in the 1940s, this weight was determined by the height and weight tables in your doctor's office. They offered a heavier ideal weight for large-framed women than for medium-framed women (which is larger than the ideal for small-framed women). For most of us, it was difficult to look at these tables without concluding we must be large-framed.

According to these ideal height and weight tables (which have been criticized for being methodologically flawed and have been abandoned by researchers),[10] an average-height woman (five feet, five inches tall) should weigh between 117 and 130 pounds if she is small-framed and from 137 to 155 pounds if she is large-framed.[11] The problem was, obese people tended to start diets weighing well above these somewhat unrealistic ideal ranges, and they rarely lost enough weight to reach them. Eventually researchers and physicians realized this, and they did the only thing they could do to increase the number of successful dieters: they changed the definition of success to one that was easier to achieve, which was losing 40 pounds. It's like a pole-vaulter lowering the bar when he realizes he cannot leap over it where it is.

According to an influential review from the 1950s, however, 95 percent of dieters failed to achieve this standard as well.[12] The response from the medical community was simply to lower the bar again. So for the next several decades, a diet that resulted in weight loss of 20 pounds was considered a success.[13] Of course, a 20-pound weight loss means something very different to a 300-pound man than it does to a 100-pound girl, and in the 1970s, researchers quite sensibly started describing weight-loss goals in relation to a person's starting weight (and later included a person's height in the calculation as well). Stated in these terms, losing 10 percent of one's starting weight was considered a successful diet. Only about 20 percent of dieters manage to achieve that goal, though,[14] and in 1995, the Institute of Medicine lowered the bar again. They decided that the goal of weight loss programs would be to lose 5 percent of one's starting weight,[15] which is just 10 pounds for a 200-pound person. At this point, our pole-vaulter probably no longer needs the pole to clear the bar.

Although researchers have continually lowered their standards, dieters have not lowered theirs. Not one dieter in a survey of 130 dieters said he would be satisfied with a 5 percent weight loss, and only one said he would be satisfied with a 10 percent weight loss.[16] Heartbreaking evidence of dieters' high (and unfulfilled) standards comes from a study that surveyed sixty obese women about their weight loss goals when they started a new diet, and then checked in with them a year later to see how much weight they lost.[17] When they were surveyed before the diet, the women selected their goal weight for the diet, and then listed their dream weight, their acceptable weight (defined as a weight they could accept, even though they would not be happy with it), and a weight that would be considered their disappointed weight—one that they "could not view as successful in any way," although less than their current weight.

The women started the diet weighing an average of 218 pounds, and their goal was to lose more than 70 pounds. They defined their acceptable weight loss as losing 55 pounds, and said they would be disappointed if they lost less than 38 pounds. In fact, the women on this diet lost an average of 36 pounds, making this an incredibly successful diet compared to the ones I summarized earlier (which averaged a 15-pound weight loss). But despite the comparative success of these women, very few were satisfied with the outcome. As shown in Figure 1, none of the women achieved the weight those height and weight tables would have defined as ideal back in the 1940s (that's why there's no bar there), none achieved her dream weight, and only 9 percent achieved their goal

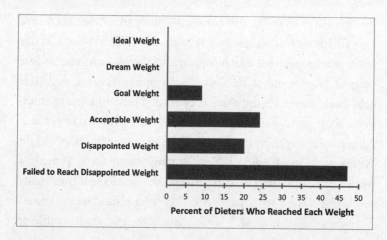

FIGURE 1. Percent of dieters reaching their ideal weight, dream weight, goal weight, acceptable weight, disappointed weight, and none of those weights.

weight. Twenty-four percent of the women achieved their acceptable weight, and 20 percent achieved their disappointed weight. That means that 47 percent of the women—nearly half—did not even lose enough weight to reach their disappointed weight.

That's the first reason why we can't say that diets work. Although people nearly always lose enough weight for researchers to consider the diet successful, they rarely lose enough weight to satisfy themselves. The second reason why we can't say diets work is that dieters do not keep off the weight that they lose.

DO DIETS WORK IN THE LONG TERM?

For most dieters, the goal is not to lose weight temporarily, nor is it to remain on a strict diet their entire life. Yet for much of the last century, researchers focused primarily on the results from the first three to six months of diets—the part of the diet where a small amount of weight is lost relatively quickly—but did not track participants for much longer. Do dieters continue to lose weight? Does some of the lost weight return? Do some dieters gain back more weight than they lost? These important questions about diets have not been examined in most diet studies. Perhaps not surprisingly, commercial diet companies like Weight Watchers, Jenny Craig, or Nutrisystem, which could provide a wealth of information on their clients' weight changes over many years, claim they are unable to collect long-term data on the effectiveness of their diets.[18] Which raises the question: unable or unwilling?

In the 1990s, when the Federal Trade Commission (FTC) began to increase its scrutiny of the weight loss industry's marketing practices, it asked a panel of experts to create guidelines for advertising weight loss products. This expert panel included representatives from several commercial diet programs, and those representatives insisted that advertisements should not have to include information about the effectiveness of a program. They said they would not offer data on the efficacy of their diets in the short term or the long term, or even the number of people who completed their programs after starting them,[19] which are pretty much the exact facts potential customers would want to know.

The representatives of the diet programs gave amazingly unconvincing reasons for why they should not have to provide this information. First, they argued that it was too costly and difficult to collect such information, even though many of them already had the information on hand. Second, they said dieters don't need this information because they have had lots of experience with diets and are already very knowledgeable about them. Their third argument, however, was the most illuminating. They said, as recorded in the FTC report, "Dieters will be discouraged if they are provided with realistic outcome data."[20] This was nothing less than an admission that their programs were not effective. The diet companies won the battle—they still do not have to disclose any of this information in their ads. But their unwillingness to report on whether their diets are effective makes it clear that they do not have much confidence in their diets, and they don't want you to know it.

If their products were effective in leading to long-term weight loss, of course, they would soon put themselves out of business. These companies count on repeat customers for their very existence. Richard Samber, the longtime financial chairman of Weight Watchers, likened dieting to playing the lottery. "If you don't win, you play it again. Maybe you'll win the second time."[21] When asked how the business could be successful when only 16 percent of customers[22] maintained their weight loss, he said, "It's successful because the other 84 percent have to come back and do it again. That's where your business comes from."[23] And come back they do. As stated in Weight Watchers' business plan, "Our members have historically demonstrated a consistent pattern of repeat enrollment over a number of years. On average . . . our members have enrolled in four separate program cycles."[24] Clearly, if long-term weight loss were achieved, their members would not need to reenroll.

The Evidence

Although diet studies have been published regularly in the scientific literature since the 1920s, very few long-term follow-up studies of diets were conducted before the 1990s, and not many have been published since then.[25] Tracking dieters in the years after a diet ends is crucial, because what happens after a diet ends, as most dieters know, is that the lost weight returns. The more time that passes, the more weight is regained. In one study, for example, a group of obese people volunteered to be starved (in a hospital) for about thirty-eight days.[26] After the starvation period, they were tracked for varying lengths of time. Among those who were followed for less than two years, 23 percent gained back more weight than they had lost. Among those who were followed for two or more years, 83 percent gained back more weight than they lost.

Even in the studies that track people for the longest periods of time (four or five years), the amount of weight regained doesn't appear to level off.[27] This is important, because it suggests that if people were followed for even longer, they may be found to have kept gaining weight. Researchers imply that their participants' weight at the end of a study is the most they'll weigh, but the end of a diet study simply means that researchers will no longer see how much more weight participants gain—it doesn't mean that participants will stop gaining weight.

To find out how effective diets are in the long term, the graduate students in my Psychology of Eating seminar and I decided to track down every study that followed dieters for at least two years after a diet began. During class discussion one day, we had concluded that what really mattered about diets was *keeping* the weight off, not just *taking* the weight off, and we were curious to find out what the research showed. We assumed there would be many articles that reviewed the research on this topic, because no matter how esoteric or narrow the research question, a paper reviewing it always seems to already exist. In this case, with such a straightforward, obvious (to us), and important question, in a field with huge amounts of research, we were shocked to find that there was no such review. So we did it ourselves. Had we known what a massive undertaking this seemingly simple project would be, we probably would have convinced ourselves not to bother. Being naive about the research on dieting, we went for it.

Most diet studies are conducted by researchers who have a vested interest in a particular outcome. I'm not saying that diet researchers would purposely tilt their findings toward showing diets work, but despite one's best intentions, bias does creep into research.[28] It's true for all of us researchers all of the time, so not having a preference for any particular outcome in this project helped us in our effort to look at the research as objectively as possible.

We hunted through the research for studies that tracked participants for at least two years after they started a diet, and that used the gold standard research design, called a randomized controlled trial. This kind of study assigns participants to either be put on a diet right away, or be wait-listed to go on the diet sometime in the distant future. The researchers can then compare the results of these two groups over time.

The crucial factor that separates randomized controlled trials from other kinds of studies is that neither the participants nor researchers have any control over whether participants are assigned to the diet or to the wait list. It is done randomly. Although it may seem counterintuitive, this makes the groups as *similar* to each other as possible. If participants picked their groups, those who were most motivated and eager to diet would select the diet condition, and those less interested would put themselves on the waiting list. It wouldn't really be fair to compare these two groups to each other, because they would each start out with different kinds of people.

There are many hundreds of diet studies, but even with six of us hunting through them thoroughly, we were able to find only twenty-one studies that satisfied our criteria.[29] The diets in these studies varied from 800-calorie-a-day "very low calorie diets" to low calorie, low fat, low carbohydrate, or combinations of these, and several also included other dietary changes such as reduced sodium, reduced cholesterol, or reduced alcohol. Some diets featured support services as well, such as group counseling or weekly phone calls.

The studies we looked at ranged from two to ten years (lasting an average of 3.6 years), and we found that at the end of that time, dieters had managed to keep off, on average, a measly two pounds.[30] Nearly half of the participants, or about 40 percent, actually weighed *more* at the follow-up than before they went on the diet. Obesity researchers know that dieters keep off only a small amount of weight, but they justify these small weight losses by suggesting that these individuals would surely have gained lots of weight if they had not participated in the diet. That's a perfectly reasonable possibility to consider. The type of study we required in our review, the randomized controlled trial, is set up to test that very question, and we found that this was clearly not the case. Participants in the no-diet conditions of these studies gained an average of just one pound. Dieters went through all that effort and self-denial, and in the end they weighed only the tiniest bit (three pounds) less than the non-dieters.[31]

Now for the really bad news. The truth is, most diets are probably even less successful than these gloomy findings suggest. The results I just described almost certainly inflate the success of these diets. Despite using the gold standard of research design, these studies have three serious flaws—flaws that are mostly unavoidable—that tilt them toward showing that diets work.[32] Each of these flaws adds to the false impression that people can keep off the weight they lose.

The first of these flaws is that the people who start and finish these studies are not necessarily typical dieters. Many people who volunteer to participate in weight loss studies are rejected from participating before the study begins. In some studies, for example, researchers only allow people to join if they are able to diet successfully in a "tryout" period for a month or more before the study starts.[33] In those cases, the people who struggle the most with dieting don't even make it into the studies. It's like giving a class a test but not letting the D and F students participate. Your class average will look impressive, but only because you have excluded those who would have scored the lowest.

That's not the only reason participants are different from typical dieters. Many of the people who do make it into studies do not stick around for the full duration of the study. They often stay on the diet for the first six to twelve months, but then do not return for the follow-up measures a year or two after that. In essence, they drop out. In these studies, an average of about 20 percent of participants dropped out.[34]

Dropping out of diet studies is so common that researchers have carefully studied the question of how dropouts might change the results. For example, researchers have compared participants who returned to be weighed two years after a diet started to those who did not, and found that the people who returned had lost more weight[35] and kept it off longer[36] than people who did not return. It seems logical, doesn't it? Imagine if you had been a part of a diet study a few years ago and had regained a lot of the weight you lost. Wouldn't it be tempting to ignore the researchers' request to come back and be weighed? You might feel embarrassed about regaining the weight and probably wouldn't be eager to face them. This is understandable, but we do need to acknowledge that studying only the people who get selected for a diet study and finish the diet gives a false impression of what happens to most people on diets. It makes diets seem more effective than they are.

The second serious flaw with these studies is that most of the participants are not weighed *in person* by the researchers at the end of the study. Instead, they weigh themselves and communicate their weight to researchers over the phone or by email. Over half of the dieters in the studies we analyzed reported their weight instead of being weighed by researchers in a lab.

This is problematic partly because people may take a guess at their weight rather than weighing themselves, or weigh themselves with an inaccurate scale. Even if they use a highly accurate scale, they still may not admit their true weight to the researchers. People tend to say they weigh less than they do. This has been documented in several studies in which researchers ask people their weight over the phone, and then—surprise!—show up on their doorstep with a scale soon after. When they compare what people said they weighed to the number on the scale, they found that, on average, non-obese people report that they weigh about five pounds less than they do, and that obese people say they weigh about eight pounds less than they do.[37] Remember that the participants in the diet studies (most of whom were obese) only maintained a weight loss of about two pounds. If they actually weighed eight pounds more than they reported to researchers, it is possible the average weight change was a six-pound weight *gain*, rather than the two-pound loss.

The third flaw in these studies is that 20 percent to 65 percent of participants went on at least one other diet while the original diet was being studied. This makes it appear as if the original diet had led to sustained weight loss, when, in fact, any weight loss is almost certainly attributable to the beginning stages of another diet. The weight hasn't stayed off; it's been regained and then lost all over again. In one of the studies, participants reported that they didn't go on another diet until they had gained back *all* the weight they lost on the diet that was being studied.[38] And in another, the researchers stated that if they had not taken into account what participants weighed when they started an additional diet, they would have falsely concluded that the diet they were studying had worked.[39] Because nearly all studies fail to take this behavior into account, diets end up looking more effective than they are.[40]

Without taking these flaws into account, the most rigorous diet studies find that about half of dieters will weigh more four to five years after the diet ends than they did at the start of the diet. This conclusion must, unfortunately, be considered a low estimate of how many people's diets will fail, since it comes from studies so strongly biased toward showing that diets work. The true number of people who fail on diets is probably much higher.

The fact that diets don't lead to long-term weight loss isn't news to diet researchers. In 1991 researchers stated that "it is only the rate of weight regain, not the fact of weight regain that appears open to debate."[41] Ten years before that, another researcher pointed out that "If 'cure' from obesity is defined as reduction to ideal weight and maintenance of that weight for 5 years, a person is more likely to recover from most forms of cancer than from obesity."[42] Researchers have known for a long time that diets don't work. Now you know it, too.

CHAPTER 2

WHY DIETS DON'T WORK: BIOLOGY, STRESS, AND FORBIDDEN FRUIT

I've given you the bad news: diets fail in the long run. Now, let's try to understand why.

In social psychology we often say that if you find that most people behave in the same way, then the explanation for their behavior has very little to do with the kind of people they are. It has to do with the circumstances in which they find themselves. For example, most students in class raise their hands and wait quietly to be called on before speaking. It's not that they are all timid or overly polite types of people. It's that the classroom setting is sufficiently powerful that without really thinking about it, nearly everyone ends up following the same unwritten rules. When we think about people who regain weight after dieting, it's a similar principle. It's not that they have a weak will or lack discipline, or that they didn't want it enough, or didn't care. It's about the circumstances in which they find themselves, and the automatic behavior that is provoked by those settings. In other words: if you have trouble keeping weight off, it is not a character flaw.

When it comes to keeping weight off, a combination of circumstances conspires against you. Each one on its own makes it difficult, but put them together and you are no longer in a fair fight. One circumstance that makes things hard is our environment of near-constant temptation (we'll talk more about this in Chapter 3). Two others are biology and psychology. I realize it may seem odd to you that I am calling these things "circumstances," but, like a classroom setting and the behavior it produces, we need to acknowledge the context in which you regain weight.

To an important extent, weight regain after a diet is your body's evolved response to starvation. When you are dieting, it may feel as though you are about to starve to death, but you know that you can open the fridge at any time and find more to eat, if you really wanted to. Your body doesn't know this, however, and you have no way to tell it that you just want slimmer hips or a flatter stomach. All your body knows is that not enough calories are coming in, so it kicks into survival mode. From an evolutionary perspective, the bodies that were best able to survive in times of scarcity (and then pass their genes on to future generations) were those that could use energy efficiently in order to get by on tiny amounts of food. Another quality that would have helped you survive was psychological: a single-minded pursuit of more fuel—and once you located it, the overwhelming urge to eat lots of every type of food you found.

Together, these biological and psychological forces make regaining lost weight all too easy. Let's take a closer look at the biological ones first, because they set the stage for everything else.

YOU CAN (PARTLY) BLAME BIOLOGY

Your genes play an important role in determining how much you weigh throughout your life. In fact, your genetic code contains the blueprint for your body type and, more or less, the weight range that you can healthily maintain. Your body tends to stay in that range—which I will refer to as your set weight range—most of your adult life. If your weight strays outside it, multiple systems of your body make changes that push you back toward it. While this may seem controversial—aren't we all in control of our own weight?—the role of your genes in regulating weight is backed up by solid evidence. And we don't even need to rely on high-tech gene mapping to understand this; we just need to study people who share the same genetics.[1]

One classic study compared the weight of more than 500 adopted children with that of their biological parents and that of their adoptive parents.[2] Obviously, if genes matter more to weight than does environment, the children's weight should be similar to the weight of their biological parents. If learned eating habits have more of an impact on weight, their weight should be more like their adoptive parents. In fact, researchers found that the children's weight correlated strongly with the weight of their biological parents and not at all with the weight of their adoptive parents.

That evidence always blows me away, but if that's not persuasive enough for you, there's also evidence from studies of twins. Twin studies are commonly used to see how much genes matter in all sorts of human features, from personality traits to psychological disorders to physical diseases. The problem for eating studies is, while identical twins share all of the same genes, they also typically share the same eating environment. So if features are common in both twins, it is possible that they are the result of a shared environment.

To tease apart the effects of genes from the effects of the shared environment, researchers located identical twins that were raised in separate homes without knowing each other. It may seem surprising that there are enough sets of twins that meet this criteria, but there are. This type of twin research was partly pioneered in the very psychology department in which I work, at the University of Minnesota (coincidentally located in the twin cities of Minneapolis and St. Paul). If you go up to the fifth floor, the walls are covered with photographs of identical twins that were separated at the age of five months (on average) and had been apart for about thirty years before being reunited as adults. The visible similarities are remarkable, as are the many documented behavioral similarities.[3]

The crucial twin study of body weight (which comes from the Swedish Adoption/Twin Study of Aging) included 93 pairs of identical twins raised apart (and 154 pairs of identical twins raised together). Sure enough, the weights of identical twins, whether they were raised together or apart, were highly correlated. That study, along with several others, led scientists to conclude that genes account for 70 percent of the variation in people's weight.[4] Seventy percent! What is truly remarkable is that this is only slightly lower than the role genes play in height (about 80 percent of the variation).[5] Don't get me wrong. I'm not saying you can't influence your weight at all, just that the amount of influence you have is fairly limited,[6] and you'll generally end up within your genetically determined set weight range.

Okay, so maybe you can't easily influence your weight to achieve long-lasting losses, you might say, but it seems all too easy to influence it in the direction of weight gain, right? Actually, it's not as easy as you might think. Researchers have studied that side of the equation, too—instead of having people *lose* weight and then try to maintain the *thin* weight, they had people *gain* weight and then try to maintain the *fat* weight. Staying fat shouldn't be that difficult, should it? In one set of studies, researchers tried to make people fat by overfeeding them. They didn't want exercise to get in the way of weight gain, so they did these studies with people they could prevent from doing any exercise at all: prisoners.[7] I'm not wild about using prisoners in research because it is often hard for them to refuse to participate, but the researchers explained their plans fully and got permission from each prisoner.

Several fascinating things happened next. First of all, it was remarkably difficult to make the prisoners fat. The prisoners had to eat enormous quantities of food—some of them over 10,000 calories per day, for four to six months—to gain 20 percent of their starting weight. That's a lot of extra calories, considering men in the United States tend to average about 2,500 daily calories. Some of the prisoners could not gain that much weight, despite eating huge amounts of food, and the prisoners gained much less weight than the researchers predicted based on the amount of calories they consumed. And most surprising, once the prisoners had gained weight, it was very difficult for them to keep it on. They had to continue eating a large number of calories per day (at least 2,700) just to maintain it; otherwise they would lose the weight. When researchers tried the same study with dedicated student volunteers who were free to walk around and exercise some, they were actually *unable to turn them obese*.[8] In another study, researchers fed twins an additional 1,000 calories per day over what they would need to eat to maintain their weight. They did this for 100 days. Like the prisoners, these twins were unable to maintain the higher weights.[9]

In addition to showing why it is so difficult to maintain a weight higher or lower than is dictated by our genes, these kinds of studies also offer evidence that our genes control *how much* weight we gain. Even when study participants were fed the same amount of calories, they gained varying amounts of weight. The pairs of twins that were overfed 1,000 calories per day gained anywhere from 9 to 29 pounds. In other words: the same number of calories led some people to gain three times as much weight as other people. Moreover, each twin gained nearly the same amount as their own twin, even though each pair of twins gained different amounts of weight than the other pairs of twins.[10] All of these studies are evidence that your body is trying to keep you within that genetically determined set weight range.[11] When our weight is within this range, we don't have to fight to maintain it. It's easy. We can eat a little more or a little less, exercise a little more or a little less—and it won't have much of a lasting impact. The hard part is trying to get out of that range, because to do so, you have to battle biology. Your body uses many biological tricks to defend your set range, particularly if you get below it, because this is when your body thinks you are starving to death. To save you, it makes you eat more food, and stores some of the energy you consume in case of emergency.

When you are dieting and hungry, your brain responds differently to tasty-looking food than it does when you are not dieting. The areas of the brain that become unusually active make you more likely to notice food, prompt you to pay more attention to it when you find it, and make it look even more delicious and tempting than usual.[12] These are potent signals to eat. At the same time, activity is reduced in the prefrontal cortex, the "executive function" part of the brain that helps you make decisions and resist impulses.[13] Either one of those responses would make you more likely to indulge, but when you put them together, you don't stand a chance. Your ability to resist is taking a snooze exactly when you most want its support. To make matters worse, this response has been found to be particularly strong in obese people—and it also gets stronger the longer you diet.[14]

Another way your body defends your set range is through hormonal changes. As you diet and lose weight, you lose body fat.[15] Many of us think of body fat as blubbery stuff that just sits there under our skin and makes us look fat, keeps us warm, and helps us float in the ocean, but body fat (also called adipose tissue) is an active part of the endocrine system.[16] It produces hormones that are involved in the sensations of hunger and fullness, and as you lose body fat, the amount of these hormones circulating in your body changes. The levels of hormones that help you feel full (including leptin, peptide YY, and cholecystokinin) decrease. The levels of hormones that make you feel hungry (including ghrelin, gastric inhibitory polypeptide, and pancreatic polypeptide) increase.[17] Just like with the changes in brain patterns, these hormone changes give you an urge to eat, and to eat a lot. One study found that these changes in hormone levels were still detectable in people a year after they stopped dieting.[18]

While these changes in brain reactivity and hormone production are pushing you to eat more, your metabolism also betrays you. It changes partly because you are thinner, and partly due to the effects of (what it perceives to be) starvation. Whether or not you are dieting, your metabolism is affected by your weight. It takes energy to run all of the metabolic processes in your body every day; the more you weigh, the more energy (calories) your body burns just to keep you alive. When you lose weight, even if starvation has no effect on your metabolism, your body will still burn fewer calories, simply because it is now a smaller body to run. This means that the number of calories you ate to lose weight eventually becomes too many calories to eat if you want to *keep* losing weight.[19]

On top of that, starvation also has an effect on your metabolism. Because there is not enough food coming in, your metabolism slows down to conserve energy. Unfortunately, this doesn't make you feel full longer or help you lose weight. Quite the opposite. It uses each calorie in the most efficient manner possible, which allows your body to run on even fewer calories than it would need just based on the size of the body. More calories are left unused and can be stored as fat.

The consequences of these changes are problematic, to say the least. When you aren't taking in enough calories, your body makes storing those calories as fat the top priority, regardless of the dietary fat content of whatever you ate.[20] That's right, in certain cases, even non-fat foods can get stored as fat. And more alarmingly, this means that a person who loses weight to reach 150 pounds, for example, is not the same, physiologically, as a person who normally weighs 150 pounds.[21] To maintain 150 pounds after dieting down to that weight, dieters must eat fewer calories per day than people who were 150 pounds all along (not to mention fewer calories per day than they ate to get to that weight) or else they will gain weight.[22]

You know what I find the most infuriating about this situation? People will blame the weight regain on your self-control, even though you are probably eating less food than they are! To maintain your new weight, you have to fight evolution. You have to fight biology. You have to fight your brain. You have to fight your metabolism. These are the ways your body tries to protect you from starvation, and it is not a fair fight. You have to respect this miracle of being human, but you don't have to like it.

SAVE SOME OF THE BLAME FOR PSYCHOLOGY

The other foe in the long-term weight loss battle is psychology. When people are dieting and hungry, psychological changes take place. We learned about a lot of these changes from a ground-breaking semi-starvation study that was conducted in the 1940s by Ancel Keys, a professor in the School of Public Health at the University of Minnesota.[23] In it, thirty-six men volunteered to be starved for six months as a humanitarian act so that researchers could test the best ways to help starving people throughout the world. Although this study is always referred to as a starvation or semi-starvation study, I think of it as a diet study, because the men were allowed nearly 1,600 calories per day.

All sorts of things happened to the men during the study, which I will talk more about later, but the most common *psychological* response was an obsession with food. Before the study started, the men had many interests. They actively followed current events; they were curious about the new city they were living in; and they wanted to become acquainted with each other. Some of them even signed up to take classes on campus. But when the men were starving, the only thing they wanted to think about, or could think about, was food. They lost interest in their humanitarian mission, stopped attending classes, and even lost interest in sex. Their conversations with each other centered on food, their dreams were about food, and their spare time was occupied with thoughts of wonderful meals they had in the past, or plans for what they would eat someday in the distant future. Several of the volunteers vowed to take up careers in the food industry when the study ended—to open a grocery store or restaurant, become a chef, or work on a farm. Even those who had never cooked before started clipping recipes and reading cookbooks (including one volunteer who collected more than twenty-five cookbooks).[24]

This type of behavior would have been useful for our ancestors during times of starvation. Individuals who focused exclusively on food and how to access it would have been more successful at finding some and, therefore, would be more likely to survive than their peers who were able to distract themselves from thoughts of food. But today, it just means that the less we try to eat, the more obsessed we become with food.

To take a closer look at this phenomenon, a collaborator[25] and I examined what happens when people are denied a particular kind of food. We asked the students in my research methods class to participate, and they roped their friends into helping us, too. We had them record how many times they thought about a particular food, every day for three weeks. One of those weeks they were told they were forbidden from eating that food. Sure enough, they thought about the food more often that week than either of the other weeks.[26] This shouldn't come as a big shock. One of the first stories in the Bible is of Eve struggling not to eat the forbidden fruit. What is surprising, though, is that unlike Eve's fixation on that delicious, tantalizing apple, the students thought about an off-limits food more frequently even if it was a food they didn't like very much.

The problem for diets is that almost by definition, you have to forbid yourself from eating all sorts of foods, and for a period longer than a week. On a diet, you will think more about food in general, because you are hungry, and you will especially think about the very foods you have forbidden yourself from having. This just makes the job of avoiding and resisting those foods even harder.

ONE MORE THING TO BE STRESSED ABOUT

There are biological reasons why you regain lost weight, and there are psychological reasons why you regain lost weight. And then there is stress, which combines both of these forces in a uniquely powerful way. You probably don't need me to define stress. It's one of those "I can't define it but I know it when I see it" sorts of things. But when psychologists talk about stress, we are referring to a negative emotional response that leads to a specific set of physical, cognitive, and behavioral changes.[27] These changes are thought to have evolved to help us handle one particular form of stress—stress that comes on suddenly and needs a quick, powerful mobilization of energy, such as fleeing from a woolly mammoth or other fast-moving predator.[28] But that is not the kind of stress we routinely encounter in our day-to-day life. The kinds of stressors we experience don't start and end quickly or suddenly. They tend to be ongoing, such as chronic worry over our finances, our jobs, or our families.

Among the physical changes that stress initiates is the release of a hormone that you've probably heard about if you've ever tried to lose weight: cortisol. This particular hormone has made headlines for its link to belly fat. That's because one of the many things cortisol does to help you flee the mammoth is to make energy—in the form of glucose—available for use in your bloodstream. But if the cause of your stress isn't chasing you across the tundra, this newly available glucose isn't needed to combat the stress right away. Instead it ends up getting stored in your belly, as fat.[29] So on a chemical level, stress causes weight gain.

Stress also leads people to act in ways that cause weight gain. Studies have shown that stress causes us to overeat,[30] exercise less, and sleep less. It is no surprise that eating more and exercising less leads to some weight gain, but many people underestimate the role of sleep when it comes to weight maintenance. Your brain responds to sleep deprivation in a similar way as it responds to hunger, even if you aren't hungry. If you are sleep deprived, even for one night, the sight of enticing food elicits a stronger-than-normal response in a part of your brain that motivates eating, and a weaker-than-normal response in the prefrontal cortex, that area of your brain that controls impulsive behavior.[31] In one sleep study, when participants were allowed to sleep only for five hours a night, they gained about two pounds in five days. But when they were allowed to sleep for nine hours a night, they had no trouble maintaining their weight over five days.[32]

So, let's think about this: Stress leads to weight gain. Most of us consider ourselves to be under stress at various points in our lives, but what about dieters? While many people on a diet will tell you that dieting is stressful, is it accurate to say that the act of dieting alone promotes a stress response?

For her dissertation, my brilliant student Janet Tomiyama set out to see if dieting actually causes that physiological chain reaction that is part of the stress response.[33] If it did, she also wanted to know what exactly about dieting was causing the problem. There are two main rules you have to follow on any diet: you have to restrict what you eat, and you have to monitor your food intake. Restricting what you eat means that you can't always have the things you want, that you have to politely say "no" when someone offers you a slice of cake at a birthday party, and that you often feel hungry. Monitoring your food intake means that you have to keep careful track of what you eat, count calories, and plan meals. These tasks could be considered stressful, or at least a giant hassle.

Janet sought out women who wanted to start a diet, and then she had her study participants restrict their calories, monitor their eating, both, or neither. Specifically, she had them restrict their eating to 1,200 calories a day and also monitor their eating by keeping a daily food diary. One group had to restrict their eating to 1,200 calories a day but *not* monitor their eating. (That part was tricky—how do you get people to eat exactly 1,200 calories without tracking their calories? For those women, Janet provided 1,200 calories a day of prepackaged food, so they didn't need to keep track of anything.) Another group had to monitor their eating by keeping a daily food diary, but they were not asked to restrict their eating to 1,200 calories. And some of the women weren't required to do any of these things.

Because Janet was interested in whether dieting caused a physiological stress response, she needed to measure the cortisol in the dieters' saliva. To do that, the women would need to provide saliva samples six times a day for a few days before and after the diet. Whenever it was time for them to give a saliva sample, they had to chew on a cotton pad called a Salivette until it was totally saturated with saliva, and then spit the whole soggy thing into a little plastic tube. It's a bit icky, but the women in the study were troupers and did this without complaint.

Until Janet could test the samples, they needed to be kept frozen. Janet ran half of the study in my old lab at the University of California, Los Angeles, and Jeff Hunger, my lab manager at the time, ran the other half in my new lab in Minnesota. Our regular freezer was full of ice cream for another study, so we acquired a special freezer solely for storing saliva samples. Rules of scientific conduct require that things researchers intend to serve people to eat may not occupy the same freezer as samples of human bodily fluids (which is not a bad rule of thumb for home freezers, either). Once the freezer was full of saliva, Jeff packed all those tubes of Salivettes in dry ice and shipped them to Janet in Los Angeles; she then did whatever one does with saliva samples to test them for cortisol (a part of the process I leave to the experts).

What Janet found is that whether or not her subjects monitored their calorie intake, the act of restricting calories led to a physiological stress response.[34] This was the first human study to prove that diets are stressful (though around the same time it was shown in mice).[35] I think its findings add an important wrinkle to how we think about dieting. It's not just that people should try to avoid stress while dieting. It's that stress *cannot be avoided when you are dieting*, because dieting itself causes stress. Dieting causes the stress response that has already been shown to lead to weight gain.

Remember, this stress response is just one of the many biological and psychological changes that happen when we restrict our eating. Each one on its own creates an obstacle to keeping off weight. Perhaps you can surmount one of these obstacles, or even two, for a while. But all of them, all of the time? It is unrealistic to expect people to succeed when they are up against evolution, biology, and psychology. It's time to try something different.

MEET YOUR NEW BEST FRIEND: YOUR SET WEIGHT RANGE

Any time I talk to people about the idea of a genetic set weight range, they focus on the bad news—that if they lose so much weight that they fall below their set range, they will probably gain it back. But don't forget about the good news. As we learned from the study of the prisoners who were purposely overfed, it is harder to gain a lot of weight than people realize. (It can happen, though, so I wouldn't recommend trying this one at home.) If you gain a lot of weight so that you are above your set range, you have to consume more calories to maintain it than someone who was that weight all along, or you will lose weight. Many people monitor their eating carefully and believe that if they didn't, they would gain a lot of weight. They are probably wrong. They would likely gain weight, but not enough to drastically change them.

So how do you determine your set range? It's more of an art than a science, at least given the current state of knowledge, but we do know that it will encompass the weights you tend to be at when you are not dieting and not engaging in extreme overeating. If there is a particular weight that you seem to keep coming back to after changes in either direction, it might be in the middle of your set range. One expert says that you can comfortably lose about fifteen pounds[36] below your set point before your body starts trying to defend a higher weight. (Of course that assumes you weigh enough to begin with—if you weigh 100 pounds, losing 15 pounds is almost certainly outside your set range.) If it works the same on the high end as on the low end, that would mean that your set range reasonably covers about thirty pounds.

Unless you want to battle evolution, biology, and psychology and be hungry every single day of your life, I wouldn't suggest trying to live below your set range. I understand that for many people, the goal is simply to be thin, but you also want to enjoy your life. Losing some weight but staying within your set range is a healthy goal; getting so thin that you are below this range is a very difficult and self-defeating one. For most of us, the aim should be to live at the low end of our set range. We'll call that weight our leanest livable weight, and it's perfectly reasonable to aim for it, and to make some lifestyle changes to get there.

But first, I want to talk a little bit more about what's *not* the cause of your weight regain: your inability to control yourself. Lack of willpower is not why people can't lose weight or maintain weight loss on a diet, and strong willpower is not why thin people stay thin. The idea that willpower is the key to weight control is misguided. It's time we set the record straight.

. . . .

CHAPTER 3

THE MYTH OF WILLPOWER

Life would be a lot easier if I liked sorbet. I am constantly finding myself in ice cream shops with my two sons, and if I actually liked sorbet, I would eat it. Fruity, lower-calorie, low-fat sorbet.[1] Instead, I have to try to resist ice cream, and I inevitably fail. Because I don't have enough willpower, and neither do you. Even without meeting you, I know this is true, because very few people do (and those people are probably not reading this book). The unfortunate fact is that hardly anybody has enough willpower to resist tempting foods if they are routinely confronted with them. And we *are* routinely confronted with them, because we live in an environment[2] in which the most tempting, most difficult-to-resist[3] foods (those with lots of fat and sugar) are inexpensive and readily accessible.

Dieting requires you to resist temptation every time. No exceptions. Esteemed obesity researcher John Foreyt said in *Living Without Dieting*[4] that dieting is like holding your breath. At some point, you have to breathe. When a food is present, you don't have to resist it just one time to be successful. You have to resist it an hour from now and ten minutes from now and one minute from now and one second from now. As long as the food is there, you have to resist it as often as you take a breath. And therein lies the problem.

Imagine you are a master of self-control. Nobody's perfect at anything, but suppose you are so good at self-control that you can successfully resist temptation 99 percent of the time. If a cookie is next to your desk while you are working, you have to resist that cookie every time you notice it—every time you look up from your computer. I don't know about you, but I look up after nearly every sentence I type. Or at least once a minute. Assuming that I am in the neighborhood of normal, so do you. Even with your amazing (and highly unlikely) 99 percent perfect self-control powers, on that 100th time you look up, you will reach for that cookie. It won't matter one bit that you resisted it successfully 99 times already. You get no credit for that. You won't be one bit different from people—like my nine-year-old son—who succumb the first time they see the cookie. You will have eaten the cookie; they will have eaten the cookie. Your amazing powers of self-control—your near-perfect willpower—will have gotten you nowhere.

SOME PEOPLE HAVE LOTS OF WILLPOWER, RIGHT?

It's not that different people don't have different aptitudes for self-control. We all fall somewhere on the spectrum between rampant self-indulgence and monk-like self-denial. To take an extreme example of the latter, people who suffer from the eating disorder anorexia nervosa, which is characterized by an obsessive desire to be thin, are able to harness near-perfect self-control. And while in this case their use of willpower is far from healthy, anorexics are nevertheless able to successfully resist temptation almost constantly. The same could be said for people who go on public hunger strikes. So it's not that self-control is an impossible feat. But for most people, when it comes to eating, having sufficient willpower matters a lot less than you would think.

Psychologists study self-control, and they often assess a person's level of self-control by having them fill out a questionnaire.[5] This assessment usually contains statements such as "People would describe me as impulsive"; "I am bad at resisting temptation"; and "I do many things on the spur of the moment." If these statements (and others) describe you very well, your score would indicate that your self-control ability is low. And perhaps it is. But your score on a self-control test doesn't provide the whole answer when it comes to willpower and food.

Many years ago, I gave the twenty research assistants in my lab a tedious task: I asked them to hunt down every study ever performed that included one of these self-control questionnaires. They found more than five hundred studies. Then I had them read each one to find the studies in which researchers not only had participants complete the self-control questionnaire, but also put the participants through an exercise in which they needed to use self-control. We found a grand total of twenty-six studies that fit the bill.

In one of the studies,[6] psychologists Malte Friese and Wilhelm Hofmann asked participants to try to resist some potato chips, and then they looked at whether subjects who got high scores for self-control on the questionnaire had been better able to resist the potato chips than subjects who scored low. They hadn't. When it came to resisting highly tempting food, it turned out that self-control ability didn't matter much.

But it's not that self-control has no impact at all on human behavior. On the contrary. A few years after we completed this research, another set of researchers tracked down more self-control studies and examined how well self-control ability correlated with the inhibition of various types of behavior.[7] When it came to things like schoolwork, grades, and even happiness and depression, self-control played a major role. Eating, however, was far less influenced by self-control ability than any other type of behavior they studied. In fact, self-control mattered only half as much for eating as it did for most other behaviors.[8]

Maybe you don't find these kinds of studies persuasive. After all, people are not necessarily willing to admit on a questionnaire that they are impulsive or that they cannot resist temptations. Some people may lack the self-awareness to admit these things to themselves, let alone write them on a psychologist's questionnaire. The truth is, psychologists have these same concerns about questionnaires, so whenever possible, we try to learn things about people without asking them about themselves.

When it comes to measuring self-control, a clever test called the "delay of gratification test" is often used.[9] For example, if you want to assess self-control in children, you're not going to get a very accurate answer by asking them questions about themselves or having them fill out a questionnaire. Instead, researchers leave them alone in a room with a marshmallow. The children are told that they will be given a second marshmallow if they can resist the first one until the researchers return. Otherwise they only get the one. The longer a child can resist the first marshmallow, the better his or her self-control.

One occupational hazard of being a psychologist is that you sometimes try these tests out on your friends and family. I made the tactical error of administering the marshmallow test to both of my sons when they were little. Each of them grabbed and ate the marshmallow before I could even get out of the room. This bodes poorly for their futures, as self-control ability is correlated with many measures of success and well-being later in life. For instance, the longer children resist the marshmallow, the better equipped they have been shown to be when it comes to dealing with stress and frustration ten years later.[10]

This measure of self-control also relates to their adult body mass index[11] thirty years later,[12] but importantly, the relationship is very small—even smaller than the correlation we found with the questionnaires.[13] So let's put the idea to bed, once and for all, that having sufficient willpower is the key to being thin. It just isn't. Self-control is an important quality to have for many things in life, but when it comes to body weight, it doesn't play that big a role.

SELF-CONTROL DEPENDS ON YOUR CIRCUMSTANCES, NOT YOUR ABILITY

I know what you're thinking: *Yes, but then how does that explain my mother-in-law, Trudie, who eats like a rabbit and stays so thin? She obviously has amazing self-control!* I would ask you to consider that your perception of Trudie may be flawed. Sometimes it may look like people are doing an impressive job of resisting something, when really they simply aren't tempted by it. Maybe your friends who are so good at resisting cookies are just not that into cookies. People like that are, after all, alleged to exist. It doesn't count as self-control if you didn't want the thing in the first place. My collaborator Joe Redden calls this "apparent self-control,"[14] because you look like you are controlling yourself, but you either never wanted the thing, or you are sick of the thing. Joe is an expert on getting sick of things (yes, it's possible to be an expert on that). He does studies in which he has people listen to a song they love twenty times in a row, or eat seventeen of one flavor of jelly bean, so that they get sick of it, and then he makes them like it again.

Perhaps this is obvious, but food preferences and desires matter. Like many women, I have experienced what it would be like to live with an entirely different set of preferences. It's a natural part of being pregnant. When I was pregnant with my older son, I had no interest in the kinds of foods I am usually tempted by—sweets like ice cream, brownies, and marshmallows. Instead, I wanted cucumbers, salads, and most of all, apples. Normally I have no feelings whatsoever about apples. They exist. I see them in stores. I see them representing the letter *A* in picture books. But when I was pregnant, they were objects of joy and deliciousness. I bet it's no coincidence that my son absolutely adores apples. I ate *a lot* of apples during that pregnancy. If ice cream was nearby, I would not eat it. Not because I was exercising impressive self-control over my diet (which, believe me, was not something I was trying to do while pregnant), but because I had absolutely no desire for it. It was like being plopped into someone else's mind and body for nine months, and it was eye-opening. It made me understand firsthand how some people would have no trouble resisting certain foods, while for other people it would be a struggle. It would have nothing to do with their self-control ability, and everything to do with their physiologically based preferences.

WHAT SABOTAGES WILLPOWER?

Every time I tell people that I study self-control, the first thing they do is ask for advice on how to control themselves. Actually, that's the second thing they do. The first thing they do—and tellingly, there are no exceptions to this pattern—is say something like, "Boy, I sure wish I had some more of *that*." And then they ask for advice. For years, I had no advice to offer. All I had was bad news. It slowly dawned on me that nearly every study on self-control (including most of my own, for a while) demonstrated the reasons why self-control so often fails us.

So what explains whether or not we can successfully control our behavior, if our own self-control aptitude isn't a reliable predictor? Well, there are lots of other variables that influence your ability to control yourself, and they can all be lumped into a category that I will call your *circumstances*. For example, are you distracted? Stressed? In a bad mood? In a good mood? Have you been controlling yourself all day and now you are tired? These things matter more than your self-control ability, and this is good news, because as we will soon discuss, your circumstances are things you can change.

Distraction and Multitasking

One circumstance that causes people to fail at self-control is distraction. Regular, ordinary distraction, such as watching TV while trying to have a conversation. This doesn't sound like a big deal until you take a moment to think about how often you are distracted every day.

Multitasking is the normal state of existence for most of us, rather than the occasional hurried exception. In fact, in his book *The Shallows*,[15] Nicholas Carr argues that the Internet is slowly destroying our "capacity for concentration," by training us to quickly scan and skim small pieces of information from all over the Internet, rather than focusing deeply on any one thing. Generations of children may be paying the price for this. In recent research, psychologists have found that while studying in their homes, students from middle school to college age lasted only about six minutes before getting distracted by their phones or computers.[16] Not a lot of time for deep thinking.

Long before I started the Health and Eating Laboratory, I did a study[17] on the effect of distraction on self-control of eating. In fact, it was the first eating study I ever ran, and I did it in graduate school with my classmate and close friend, Andrew Ward. The lab rooms we were given for the study were in the dingy basement of the psychology building at Stanford. It was so gloomy down there that we weren't surprised to learn that they had previously been used as prison cells in the infamous Stanford Prison Experiment in 1971.[18]

Andrew and I had found some research that showed drinking alcohol caused dieters to overeat.[19] Since we were just out of college ourselves, we knew it wasn't unusual for college students to eat piles of some crazy food after a long night of partying. At my alma mater, the University of Virginia, there is a diner called the White Spot that is famous for serving a sandwich consisting of two glazed doughnuts slapped around a scoop of ice cream, and then fried on the grill. This was (and is) notoriously eaten late at night while drunk. Overeating while intoxicated is definitely something that happens. We wanted to know *why* it happens.

We thought that maybe alcohol clouds your thinking[20] and keeps you from noticing that you are overeating. If that were true, then perhaps dieters would overeat if we clouded their thinking in another way, say by simply distracting them. Thus, our study was born. We brought students into the lab, one at a time, and asked them to eat cookies, M&Ms, and Doritos while watching a slide show of dozens of paintings. We told them that later there would be a memory test on the paintings, and that we provided the snacks to put them in a good mood so that we could study the effects of their mood on their memory. None of this was true.

In social psychology we call that a "cover story." In the regular world we call it a "lie." We believe this to be a harmless lie, and that our participants don't much care if we are studying the effects of mood on memory or the effects of distraction on eating. This type of deception is necessary in most eating research because we can't learn about people's behavior around food if they know we're observing their eating, or if they even think we might *notice* how much they're eating. When people know they're being watched, they become self-conscious, act unnaturally, and won't eat very much. So we have to be a little sneaky. We pile their bowls extremely high with food so that they can eat quite a lot without making a noticeable dent in it. And we use a cover story to explain why there happens to be an impressive spread of food there in the first place. But with every study, we are very careful to minimize the deception, and we always explain the setup to research participants at the end of the study.[21] In twenty years of conducting eating studies, we have not had a participant who seemed to be distressed by our methods.

In this study, we were interested in how much dieters and non-dieters ate when they were distracted. We could tell how much they ate because we secretly weighed the food before we gave it to them, and then weighed it again after they were done. To make sure we distracted them enough, we had them look at the slide show of paintings while listening for a tone from the computer. They were instructed to press a button on the floor as fast as they could, with their foot, every time they heard the tone. Although this seemed somewhat odd to the participants, we put the button on the floor so that their hands would be free to do what we really cared about: grab food. For comparison, we also had dieters and non-dieters who only had to listen for the tone and then hit the floor button when they heard it, without watching the slide show. Since these students are just staring at an empty wall, they shouldn't be distracted very much at all.

What we found was that the dieters who we distracted with the slide show ate about 40 percent more of the candy and chips than the dieters who we didn't distract with the slide show. Distraction interfered with their ability to control their eating. The non-dieters, on the other hand, ate about 30 percent *less* when they were distracted than when they weren't. Non-dieters' eating habits are pretty sensible, if you think about it. They are occupied with whatever is distracting them, so they don't have the time or inclination to focus on anything else, including food. This is a pattern that we notice time and time again, not just in our own work, but in that of other researchers, too.[22] Lots of everyday events cause dieters to overeat, but don't have the same effect on non-dieters.

It turned out that Andrew and I were correct in our hypothesis that clouding dieters' thoughts would lead them to overeat, but we were wrong about why it happened. We thought dieters would be so distracted that they would lose track of how much they had eaten and then inadvertently eat more than they intended. But at the end of the study, we asked dieters how much they had eaten, and they were perfectly accurate in their estimates. They hadn't lost track of their eating. We see this in lots of our studies. Dieters always know how much they ate. Are they worse at multitasking? Are they using the task as an excuse to eat? We still aren't quite sure why distraction causes them to overeat. We just know that it does.

Good Moods Can Mess You Up as Much as Bad Moods

As we've discussed, stress is one cause of dieting failure, as it is linked to both physiological and psychological changes that promote weight gain. Of course, we don't need a study to tell us that stress causes people to overeat. There's even a term for it: stress eating. And people do indeed stress eat.

But what about people on diets? If diets are a source of stress, it would seem logical that dieters would be more prone to stress eating than non-dieters, and plenty of research backs that up.[23] This was first shown in 1975, in a study[24] conducted by eating research pioneers Peter Herman and Janet Polivy. They used a complicated cover story in which their participants—who were both dieters and non-dieters—were told that they were about to receive either a painful electric shock or a very mild one. The researchers never shocked them, of course. Even back in 1975, shocking one's research participants wasn't considered an acceptable method of bringing about scientific progress. But the participants believed it, and those who were told that they were about to be administered a painful shock became quite stressed. Those who were expecting to receive a mild shock did not.

To examine the effects of stress upon eating, the researchers gave participants bowls of ice cream and measured how much they ate while waiting to be shocked. The participants who were on a diet and who were told to expect a big shock ate more ice cream than the participants who were on a diet and expecting a mild shock. Clearly, stress causes overeating, but the interesting thing about this study is, only the dieters ate more when they were stressed. Non-dieters actually ate *less* when they were stressed. Yet again, a circumstance in which we find ourselves regularly—being stressed—causes dieters to overeat but does not necessarily have the same effect on non-dieters. Not only do dieters overeat when they are stressed, but they also tend to choose foods that are particularly high in calories or fat.[25]

The amount of stress that causes dieters to lose control of their eating does not have to be as extreme as the stress of waiting to receive a painful electric shock. Much milder stressors—like watching an unpleasant movie[26]—also cause dieters to overeat. In fact, just being in a run-of-the-mill bad mood is sufficient motivation for most dieters to overeat. My student Janet Tomiyama and I learned about bad moods and eating many years ago, when we[27] studied students outside of a lab setting, as they went about their daily lives. We loaned them each a Palm Pilot (remember those?) and set it to beep once every waking hour for four days. When it beeped, they had to answer questions about their current mood and eating. We were surprised to learn that bad moods triggered eating for dieters *and* for non-dieters. But get this: so did good moods! That also surprised us at first, but once we thought about it, it didn't seem so unusual. If you're in a terrible mood and having a lousy day, you might decide to treat yourself to a doughnut. Why not? A doughnut will cheer you up (or so you think). Conversely, you are in a wonderful mood and had a productive day, and so you decide to reward your hard work with a doughnut. Why not? You deserve it!

Controlling One Thing Makes It Hard to Control Another

One reason self-control ability matters so little when it comes to eating, and circumstances matter so much, is that no matter how much willpower you may have, it is a limited resource. You can only use it for a little while before it runs out—and when that happens, it takes some time for it to replenish. Think of it like working a muscle. If you want to get strong arms and you do as many push-ups as you can, eventually your arms will start to shake and you can't go any further. That's because you have depleted the resources of those muscles. You know that you have to rest and refuel before you can use them again. Self-control isn't a muscle, but it does seem to work in much the same way. If you are relying on the strength of your willpower to control one thing, you'll be less able to exercise self-control over the next thing you encounter.

This wearing-out or depletion of self-control has been extensively documented[28] in the research literature, probably more than any other source of self-control failure. To fully appreciate it, let's consider an example.[29] Imagine you show up for a study and you are seated in a small room, with a bowl of radishes and a plate of chocolate chip cookies in front of you. The cookies are still warm and have that wonderful smell unique to freshly baked cookies. Now imagine that a researcher tells you that you are participating in an experiment about taste perception, and that you have been assigned to taste the radishes. He leaves you alone, and you have to resist the cookies and eat only radishes. This takes some self-control. Luckily, this takes only a few minutes, and with effort, you do manage to resist them for this short amount of time. This was an act of self-control. It took willpower. When the researcher comes back into the room, he takes away all of the food and asks you to help him solve a puzzle that is completely unrelated to the taste perception study. At least, that's what he says.

As you've seen in several sneaky eating studies now, things are not quite as the researcher says. Not only is this "unrelated" puzzle very much related to the study, it is also cleverly designed so that even though it looks reasonably easy, it is in fact unsolvable. Persisting at trying to solve this puzzle is an activity that requires self-control. Participants who had just resisted eating the warm cookies gave up on the puzzle very quickly, because they had just used up a large reserve of self-control. Other participants, however, had been allowed to eat the cookies during the first part of the study, so they didn't deplete their self-control resources. They persisted for longer at trying to solve the puzzle. Exercising self-control in the first task clearly reduced the subjects' ability to exercise self-control in the second task.

It is quite common to try to control two things in a row. In some sense, practically everything that you do can be considered an act of self-control, at least when it comes to the effect it has on controlling something else afterward. Hiding your emotions while watching a violent movie counts as self-control, as does trying not to think about a white bear or crossing out all the letter *e*'s in a paragraph.[30] Even such trivial (and relatively simple) acts of self-control as these led research participants to fail at controlling themselves at something else afterward.

Of course, those are not things that you do in your life (unless you happen to be a participant in one of these studies or have some very odd hobbies). But plenty of things that you do regularly engage in also mess up your ability to control something else. One of the most common of these activities is being faced with multiple choices and needing to make a decision. While nobody wants to have *no* choices in their lives, there is a downside to having too much choice.[31] My former graduate school classmate and social psychologist Sheena Iyengar conducted a study that showed that if people chose a piece of candy from a display of thirty different chocolates, they were less satisfied with the candy than if they chose from a display of only six chocolates.[32] The more choices, it seems, the greater the pressure to get it right, and the greater the possibility of feeling regret.

Making choices has been shown to deplete self-control resources, leading to worse self-control on a subsequent task.[33] This is truly unfortunate, because we make choices regularly, not just between products, but also between activities to engage in, friends to call, and recipes to make for dinner tonight. We channel-surf among 800 cable channels to select a show to watch, scroll through 1,200 songs on our smartphones to select one to listen to, and choose among millions of blogs to read and Twitter feeds to follow. Most of the time we are making a choice about something. If making a choice causes us to fail at subsequent tasks that require self-control—which it does—then we are in trouble when it comes to more than just dieting.

In fact, President Barack Obama acknowledged the burden of making choices in a 2012 *Vanity Fair*[34] interview, in which he mentioned this research and said: "You'll see I wear only gray or blue suits. I'm trying to pare down decisions. I don't want to make decisions about what I'm eating or wearing. Because I have too many other decisions to make." By limiting the number of decisions he makes, he may be helping to protect himself from making impulsive decisions. At a minimum, it keeps him from depleting his self-control resources before breakfast.

SMART REGULATION

Although we know that self-control can become depleted quite easily, we still do not know why this happens. It could be that exercising self-control makes you tired, and once tired, you lack the energy to control something else. It could be that you just get sick of controlling things, and so after controlling one thing, you can't be bothered to try again right away. It could be that controlling one thing is distracting, and as we've discussed, distraction reduces your ability to control another thing.

Not knowing why self-control becomes depleted makes it hard to come up with solutions for enhancing it. It seems that one way in which self-control is *not* like a muscle is that we can train our muscles to get stronger and work more efficiently, but we can't really train ourselves to get better at self-control. Several researchers (and a gazillion unscientific websites) claim you can "harness" your willpower abilities or learn to control yourself through a variety of exercises. These experts[35] always cite the same handful of articles,[36] but none of them actually offers convincing evidence that you can strengthen willpower like a muscle.

Humans were simply not made to willfully resist food. We evolved through famines, hunting and gathering, eating whatever we could get, when we could get it. We evolved to keep fat on our bones by eating the foods that we see, not resisting them. It is difficult to imagine how any species could evolve to be successful at resisting the foods that keep it alive. I am not saying there are not times when you would be better off resisting food. Of course there are. I am simply saying that you will not be good at it. You were not meant to be good at it.

Think of willpower as brute strength. The amount of it you need is larger than the amount of it that you have, and the amount you have is all too easily depleted by nearly everything you do. It's foolish to rely on it. In the Netherlands they say, "if you can't be strong, you must be smart,"[37] and that is the solution to the willpower problem: using your brain to make sure you don't need any.[38]

PART TWO

WHY YOU ARE BETTER OFF WITHOUT THE BATTLE

....

CHAPTER 4

DIETS ARE BAD FOR YOU

Is anyone going to disagree with me if I say that it sucks to be on a diet? I know this from personal experience, because I went on a diet once. In high school, with my girlfriends. None of us was overweight, but it seemed like the thing to do. We made up the rules ourselves, though what we based them on I cannot recall. Cheese was allowed, but milk wasn't. Bread was not allowed, but Ritz crackers and Wheat Thins were part of the daily menu. So were pickles and canned tuna fish with Miracle Whip. We had to stay below 1,200 calories each day, which is pretty standard for a diet and not nearly as strict as many. But it was miserable.

I hadn't thought very much about what I was eating before I went on the diet, then suddenly I was tracking every bite I ate and my mind was full of calorie counts. The world quickly divided into foods I could eat and foods I could not eat. I started craving foods that I typically ate infrequently, but were all the more enticing now that they were off-limits. Like doughnuts. While I was on the diet, my mom brought home a kind of doughnut that was new to me. I recall it vividly: a glazed buttermilk bar. I didn't eat it, but I was very aware that as long as I was on a diet, it would be off-limits.

My lifelong interest in *never dieting* started after just two weeks on that diet. I still remember that feeling of grayness, of life without the pleasing zing of color an occasional doughnut provided. I remember those urgent cravings for foods I hadn't found special before, and that feeling of being denied what other people got to have. No doubt many dieters will agree that my two weeks were pretty standard. I recall my father saying, "It's so hard. Nothing's harder," as he glumly packed his tiny can of fruit cocktail—his entire allotted lunch on his diet—into his briefcase to take to work. Of course we know that diets cause relatively minor miseries. I could understand enduring these miseries if diets were highly effective. I am not, after all, opposed to sacrifice for a good reason. But diets are not effective, and more important, they cause more than minor miseries—they can also cause serious problems. Plus obesity, as we will soon discuss, is not as good a reason as you think.

DIETS MESS UP YOUR THINKING

The men who volunteered for Ancel Keys's semi-starvation study[1] in 1944 definitely had a good reason to "diet." As pacifists, they were conscientious objectors to fighting in World War II, and they were eager to help those who were suffering because of it. Keys planned to starve the men for six months and then test several different refeeding menus on them, so that the safest, most effective method could be recommended to the starving troops coming back from battlefields, as well as starving populations around the world. In the process, Keys was going to learn everything he possibly could about the effects of starvation on the human body and mind.

At the time, very little was known about the biological effects of starvation, and anything that was known was gleaned from observations of the unfortunate souls who happened to find themselves in that situation. Most populations of starving people are the victims of famine or war and hardly have the ability or inclination to document their experience, but there's another category of starving people who tend to chronicle their lives meticulously: explorers. Explorers didn't always find the new lands they were searching for, and sometimes they ran out of food. But they almost always kept journals. From those journals we know that while starving, explorers were preoccupied with thoughts of food and apathetic about pretty much everything else. One member of an expedition that was unexpectedly stranded in the Arctic for an entire winter wrote, "Our constant talk is about something to eat, and the different dishes we have enjoyed, or hope to enjoy on getting back to civilization."[2] He also mentioned feeling "an apathy and cloudiness impossible to shake off."[3] We also know that starving explorers were (not surprisingly) irritable. Another member of that expedition wrote, "We are all more or less unreasonable, and I only wonder that we are not all insane. All, including myself, are sullen, and at times very surly."[4]

It's hard to know what to make of this account, or any account written by an explorer. Explorers are not your average guys, and Arctic explorers . . . Well, to be fair, I am an indoor person and cannot begin to comprehend this, but to head for the Arctic in the days before Thinsulate and electric blankets (or even electricity) is walking a fine line between brave and crazy. One explorer came so close to starving to death that he ate his boots, but instead of retiring to the tropics after being rescued, opted to go back to the Arctic.[5]

Explorers tend to also be proud, as well as on the stoic side, which might lead them to play down their suffering, even in the privacy of their journals. It's likely their symptoms were worse than they reported. It's also possible that their symptoms had little to do with starvation. If explorers were anxious, perhaps it had more to do with their concern that they might encounter a polar bear or fall off an ice floe, and less to do with hunger. It is for this reason that Keys wrote "the psychology of people exposed to 'natural starvation' is as much a psychology of fear and desperation as a psychology of hunger and food deprivation."[6] It is impossible to separate the effects of starvation from the effects of whatever traumatic situation caused the starvation in the first place.

Keys wanted to study the effects of starvation in safety and comfort, and that is exactly what he did. He created a brochure depicting impoverished children with a caption that read, "Will you starve that they be better fed?" and he distributed it at the service camps where conscientious objectors were stationed during the war. From more than four hundred men who responded, Keys selected thirty-six that he deemed physically and mentally healthy enough to take part in his study. The men moved to the campus of the University of Minnesota and lived in a special dorm under the football stadium.

For the first three months, they ate 3,500 calories per day while Keys and his staff measured everything about them. Not only the size of each body part, but also the functioning of every system of the body, from respiration and circulation to endocrine function and metabolism, plus the condition of their skin and bones, their posture, muscular abilities, sensory abilities, mental abilities, and psychological state. If it was possible to measure something, Keys measured it. These were baseline measures that would be used as a comparison for the measurements taken while the men were starving. After three months of living under these baseline conditions, the men spent the next six months on a semi-starvation diet, which was composed mainly of bread, potatoes, cabbage, and rutabagas.

The experiences of these volunteers make an interesting case study of the effects of dieting, because their semi-starvation diet provided them 1,570 calories a day. To most people these days, that does not sound like starvation at all, but rather a fairly manageable diet. But things were different back then, and this was less than half as many calories as the men were used to eating. They lost 25 percent of their body weight in six months, and pictures taken at the end of the diet show emaciated men with gaunt faces.[7] You shouldn't be surprised to learn that they regained all the lost weight, plus more, within a year of the diet ending. But along the way they experienced psychological symptoms that can reasonably be considered side effects of semi-starvation, or dieting.

The most common symptom was a preoccupation with food. As you may recall from Chapter 2, during this semi-starvation study, these men did nothing but talk and think and dream about food. In fact, the announcement of Japan's surrender, which effectively ended the war, was made while the men were eating one of their small meals. "This went through the group and we kept on eating," said one of the participants, years later. "The food was the important thing. We didn't care whether the war was over or not as long as we got our food."[8]

This intense focus on food is also evident in the journals of Arctic explorers, but for explorers, a single-minded pursuit of food is a little more practical. They needed to devote all of their mental and physical energy to finding their next meal, since they weren't sure where it would come from. But being preoccupied with food made little sense for the volunteers in the semi-starvation study. They were safely living at the university and didn't have to forage for their next meal. Nevertheless, their focus on food does not surprise me, based on my brief experience of dieting. It's remarkable how quickly thoughts of food take over when you feel deprived. And lest you think this preoccupation with food is merely a harmless nuisance, it isn't. The men in the semi-starvation study reported that they were unable to concentrate for more than a brief period of time, that they were having trouble forming thoughts, that their comprehension had declined, and that they were unable to stay alert. The formal tests of "intellective functions," as Keys called them, were quite different than tests that are used today, and not particularly sensitive to cognitive difficulties. Even still, the men performed worse on many of them during starvation, compared to the baseline period beforehand.[9]

The clearest evidence that dieting causes cognitive impairment comes from a series of laboratory experiments in which researchers asked a group of dieters and a group of non-dieters to complete the same series of mentally challenging tasks.[10] These studies have shown that dieters cannot remember as many words or sentences as non-dieters, they can't focus their attention on a task as long as non-dieters, and they react more slowly to stimuli when speed matters.[11] In addition, and most important, dieters experience impaired central executive function, that all-important aspect of cognition that is necessary for impulse control. Executive function allocates your attention to competing demands,[12] and when it is limited, it interferes with your ability to plan, make decisions, and solve problems, all of which are necessary for effective self-control.

These differences in cognitive functioning are not a biological result of malnutrition or of being underweight.[13] Instead, the impairments have been linked to that preoccupation with food thoughts[14] that was common in starving explorers, the men in Keys's study, and, it turns out, most dieters. As one lifelong dieter told me, "Thinking about diets and what I am doing wrong takes up about ninety percent of my head space." And British comedian Vanessa Engle observed, "you can be reading about Syria or Egypt, and at the same time there are these trivial but revealing thoughts in your head like, 'I shouldn't have had that for breakfast.'"[15]

Focusing extensively on food and eating (and sometimes also concerns about your weight) steals valuable attention from other activities, and the more preoccupying food thoughts dieters have, the more difficulty they experience thinking about other things and handling other cognitive tasks.[16] It doesn't take much for a dieter to become preoccupied with thoughts of food. In one study, researchers tested dieters and non-dieters on their memory ability before and after having them eat a chocolate bar. Not surprisingly, dieters had more preoccupying food thoughts after eating the chocolate bar, and their memory function suffered as a result.[17] These kinds of memory and problem-solving deficits may make it difficult for dieters to successfully focus on important daily activities.

You might be tempted to conclude that dieters are not as smart as non-dieters, which is why they struggle with thinking, remembering, planning, and problem solving. This is not true. The same studies that show cognitive impairments in dieters find no differences between dieters and non-dieters in general intelligence.[18] One of the studies compared cognitive ability in people when they were dieting and when they were not dieting, and only found that cognition was impaired when the individuals were dieting.[19] So it's not that people who go on diets aren't smart, but that dieting causes people to, in essence, be less smart than they are.

One other thinking deficit that occurs when people diet is distorted time perception. Time seems to move more slowly when you are on a diet. The men in the Keys study experienced this, and it has also been documented in studies of men who lost large amounts of weight on strict diets. Their time perception changed from before to after they lost weight.[20] Research has also found that trying to control anything at all causes this same experience of time moving more slowly.[21] I've heard it said that being on a diet doesn't make your life longer; it just makes it *feel* longer.[22] There may be more truth to this than anyone would have thought.

DIETING IS STRESSFUL

You wouldn't mind your life feeling longer if you were enjoying yourself. But time moving slowly when you're feeling bad is especially unpleasant. And when you're on a diet, you often feel bad. In particular, as Janet Tomiyama showed when she had people diet and then assayed their saliva, dieting causes a stress response, a release of the hormone cortisol into your bloodstream.[23]

In addition to making it hard to keep weight off, cortisol sets off a stream of chemical changes throughout your body. We know that cortisol's job is to get energy out of the places it's stored and make it readily accessible for you to respond to immediate stressors. In order to do that, energy gets diverted from bodily functions that aren't immediately useful for fighting or fleeing from a predator. The kinds of functions that are switched off for a bit include immune function, reproduction, growth, and energy storage. If this stress response happens every once in a while, it's no big deal. But if it happens a lot, say every time you worry about your job, your relationship, or whether you ate an inappropriate amount of marshmallow Peeps for a respectable adult, the changes it causes add up and may lead to serious physical problems.[24] Over time you become more susceptible to infections. Bone density decreases. Your blood pressure increases and blood vessels get damaged, because your heart has to work harder to divert these energy resources. The body becomes more insulin resistant and increased fat gets stored in the abdomen, which is the least healthy place to store it.

In addition to these well-documented effects of the stress response, there are some other responses to stress that scientists are only starting to get a handle on. The most exciting research on this topic, in my view, again comes from Janet and her collaborators, who have conducted studies that suggest excessive cortisol release may also harm a part of a cell responsible for aging. This part of a cell, called a telomere, is a protective cap at the end of a chromosome. Every time a cell divides, telomeres get shorter. Telomeres eventually get so short that cells can no longer divide, at which point the cells die. As this happens to more and more of your cells, the effects of aging appear—muscles weaken, skin wrinkles, eyesight and hearing fade, and thinking abilities diminish. Janet found that the more cortisol people released in response to stress, the shorter were their telomeres.[25] And other researchers have found that chronic dieters have shorter telomeres than non-dieters.[26] This work is still in its infancy, but it is possible that dieting, or the stress from dieting, may actually accelerate the aging process.

DIETS MAKE YOU FEEL BAD

We've been talking about the physical problems that may result from the stress of dieting, but let's not forget how stress feels. For many people, the unpleasant consequences of dieting are emotional ones, such as depression, low self-esteem, or even anger.[27] The starving volunteers in Keys's study experienced "general emotional instability" and became "increasingly ineffective in their daily life," as Keys wrote,[28] and six of the thirty-six volunteers had more serious psychological responses. Their symptoms included extreme mood swings, compulsive gum chewing (of dozens of packs a day, until Keys limited gum to two packs per day), shoplifting, and bouts of unrewarding cheating on the diet by eating, for example, raw rutabagas or garbage.

One of these six men had such a severe reaction that while chopping wood for a friend, he chopped three fingers off his hand with an ax. He may have done this in a desperate attempt to get kicked out of the study. The volunteers were technically free to drop out of the study at any time, but they tended to view their participation as a badge of honor, a sign of their toughness and their willingness to sacrifice for the war effort. The pressure to be virtuous certainly raised the stakes. Sure enough, this volunteer stayed in the study and adhered to the diet while in the hospital. Was it an accident? Even the man himself isn't sure. Fifty years later he remarked to an interviewer, "I still . . . am not ready to say I did it on purpose. I am not ready to say I didn't."[29]

Overall, however, severe reactions like his were atypical. Aside from the bothersome preoccupation with food, the most common problem among the men in the starvation study was depression. Is depression a typical consequence of dieting? Well, yes and no. Many studies find high levels of depression in dieters,[30] but others show improvements in mood right after a diet.[31] It's not unusual for people to begin a diet when things aren't going well in their life, so their "before dieting" mood may look pretty grim. And if you catch people about six months after starting a diet, right around when they have taken off some weight and haven't yet started regaining it, their "after dieting" mood will look pretty good. There are lots of studies set up in this way,[32] and those are the ones that show that dieting improves your mood. On the other hand, some studies measure your moods every week while you are on a diet. Those studies find that the daily process and experience of dieting causes symptoms of depression, and for many dieters, those symptoms can be severe enough for people to be diagnosed with a clinical case of depression.[33]

Even when dieting does not lead to a serious disorder like depression, it can lead to other unpleasant feelings, because dieters tend to mix up their eating habits with the emotions of guilt and shame. In fact, breaking a diet is one of the most frequent responses people give on surveys when they are asked what makes them feel guilty.[34] Dieters are much more likely than non-dieters to say they experience feelings of guilt based on food,[35] and nearly half of the women in one study agreed that they felt guilty after eating potato chips, ice cream, or candy.[36] I once turned down the free pretzels on an airplane and the stranger sitting next to me offered some unsolicited words of comfort: "You don't have to feel bad about eating those. They're low fat." As annoying (not to mention insulting) as I found her remark, this sort of comment does not violate social conventions. We—and I would argue, women in particular—are expected to feel guilt about eating.

This needs to stop. I say this as a person, not as a scientist. There is no cause for guilt or shame about things you eat. Eating is not a moral act. Perhaps there are certain circumstances in which eating can be immoral, such as the occasional act of cannibalism, taking candy from a baby, or finishing your husband's carton of salted caramel ice cream before he gets home from work. But aside from situations like those, eating or not eating a particular food should not be a source of guilt or shame. Psychologist Deb Burgard, who works with individuals with eating disorders, has an attitude the rest of us should take note of. In response to an interviewer posing a question about her guilty pleasures, she burst out laughing and said, "I don't have much use for guilt around pleasure."[37]

To be fair, guilt has its redeeming qualities. Because guilt is a negative response to a real or perceived failure,[38] it tends to motivate people to try to repair what went wrong. On certain occasions, this can be useful. The problem is when guilt starts to morph into shame. Shame occurs when instead of feeling bad about a particular mess-up, the feeling spreads to a more general sense of messing up, causing you to feel like a bad person. Shame is more painful than guilt, and to add injury to insult, shame has been shown to lead to a release of—you guessed it—the stress hormone cortisol,[39] and another kind of cell in the immune system (called a proinflammatory cytokine), which, among other things, can promote the growth of disease.[40] In addition to these physical problems, shame is also linked to psychological problems such as depression, anxiety, low self-esteem, and eating disorders.[41]

Even without the link to shame, dieting has been implicated in the development of eating disorders, although it is not clear if dieting is truly a *cause* of these disorders. On the one hand, the eating disorder of anorexia is characterized by excessive restriction of eating, so it is not possible to have it—by definition—without dieting. But to say the diet caused anorexia is perhaps unfair. On the other hand, eating disorders that are characterized by binge eating do not, by definition, have to include dieting. And yet, it is likely that individuals with binge eating disorders (including bulimia) were on a diet first.[42] The volunteers in the Keys study were prone to binge eating after the starvation ended, and many reported feeling an insatiable hunger, regardless of how much they ate, which lasted for more than a year. The results of lab experiments on this topic, however, are inconsistent,[43] and recent evidence suggests that only certain types of diets lead to binge eating. These diets involve full-on fasting,[44] or else extreme calorie restriction or meal replacement.[45] For example, reducing your calories by 50 percent seems to lead to binge eating, but reducing by 25 percent does not.[46]

If severe calorie restriction leads to binge eating, it may have something to do with neurological responses to restriction. The longer people restrict their calories, the stronger their brain responses become to images of food and to actual food.[47] This brain activity is observed in areas responsible for reward and attention, as well as craving.[48] At the same time, activity quiets down in the prefrontal cortex, the area responsible for controlling impulses. When you combine hunger from strict dieting with extra attention to food, a more positive response to food, cravings for it, and reduced self-control, it certainly sounds like a recipe for binge eating.

ONE LAST PROBLEM

Years ago I did a research project with women who were struggling with substance abuse problems, and one of the women earnestly told me that quitting heroin was easy—she'd done it five times. By that definition, dieting is easy, too. Many dieters lose the same ten or more pounds multiple times, and one dieter told me that if she lost all the pounds she's lost in her life at once, she would disappear from this earth. It's typical to lose weight, regain some or all of it, and then go on another diet. This is often referred to as yo-yo dieting. The official term for it is weight cycling, and it is common in dieters. In a study of more than 45,000 female nurses, 80 percent had dieted at least once in the previous four years, and more than half of those dieters had been on more than one diet during that time. Twenty-five percent of the dieters had lost more than ten pounds three or more times.[49]

There is no consensus in the medical community on whether weight cycling is unhealthy. Researchers can't even agree on what constitutes weight cycling. How much weight do you have to lose, how much of that do you have to regain, and in what time frame? How many times do you have to lose weight and regain it to count as a weight cycler?[50] The situation is further complicated because with many diseases, it is common for people to lose weight as they get sicker, and researchers don't always know whether people lost weight as part of an intentional diet, or if they unintentionally lost weight because they were ill.

There are some studies that show that weight cycling (with intentional weight loss) has no health consequences,[51] and a few that suggest that it's good for you,[52] but the majority of the evidence suggests that weight cycling is associated with an increased risk of illness and death.[53] Those studies find that you are better off maintaining a stable obese weight than starting obese, losing weight, and gaining it back. In one study, for example, researchers measured men's weight four times over fifteen years and categorized them according to whether they were weight cyclers. Then they looked at who lived and who died over the next fifteen years. They found that men who had weight cycled were more likely to die in that time period then men who were not obese,[54] whereas men who stayed obese the whole time lived just as long as their slimmer peers. And it doesn't appear to be the case that the men who weight cycled engaged in other unhealthy behaviors that would have increased their odds of dying.

IS DIETING REALLY WORTH THE TROUBLE?

At worst, dieting can be hazardous for your mental and physical well-being. At best, it is ineffective and unpleasant. Low-carb diets, for example, are known to cause bad breath, and a side effect of the cabbage soup diet is "almost unavoidable" gas.[55] Diet pills are another can of worms entirely. I won't go there, except to mention that the website for the diet drug Xenical includes the following among its most likely side effects: "oily rectal discharge," "passing gas with oily discharge," "urgent need to have a bowel movement," and "being unable to control your bowel movements."[56]

Those are deal-breakers to me, but none of these side effects seem to stop the millions of people who go on these diets (or use these pills). Maybe the other physical and psychological miseries of dieting I discussed here don't seem particularly troublesome to you, either. Maybe they seem like they would be worth enduring for the sake of overcoming obesity and preventing all of the many diseases it causes. But there are two problems with that logic. As you've now seen, diets don't cure obesity, and as we'll discuss next, obesity is not as bad for you as you think.

....

CHAPTER 5

OBESITY IS NOT A DEATH SENTENCE

You might be under the impression that obesity is going to kill us all. I couldn't blame you, given the headlines "Obesity bigger health crisis than hunger,"[1] or "Obesity on track as No. 1 killer."[2] You may have seen interviews with scientists who liken obesity to "a massive tsunami heading toward the United States."[3] The prevalence of obesity has increased dramatically from about 15 percent of Americans in the late 1970s to nearly 36 percent in 2010,[4] causing some scientists to suggest that the current generation of children will be the first to have shorter life spans than their parents.[5] This is scary stuff, especially coming from scientists, and you probably never thought to question it. But scientists aren't perfect and the media have a tendency to be hysterical when it comes to health headlines. So let's take a closer look at the research before we start fretting over our children's life spans.

IS OBESITY GOING TO KILL YOU?

On the first day of my health psychology course, I try to get my students excited about the possibility that psychological factors (such as stress, or their personality, or their social status) can affect their physical health. I tell them about a strange study that shows that if you are unlucky enough to have a name in which your initials spell a word with negative connotations (like "B.A.D." or "P.I.G."), you will have worse health than someone whose initials spell something with positive connotations (like "W.I.N." or "T.O.P.").[6] This link between your initials and your health suggests that psychological processes that seem like they would have nothing to do with physical health can affect it. In this case, the psychological factors might include your self-esteem, or how much of a hassle it is every time you tell someone your name and they raise an eyebrow and say, "Your parents gave you the initials P.O.O.?" The initials study suggests that those kinds of negative interactions may add up over your lifetime and affect your health.

To do that study, researchers needed to know two pieces of information about people: their full name and their health. There are many kinds of information that researchers can use to decide how healthy people are, and each type of information has certain advantages and disadvantages. None is perfect. One often-used measure, for example, is the number of sick days people take from their job. An advantage of that measure is that it can often be easily accessed from people's work records. A disadvantage is that people often take sick days for reasons other than being sick.

Part of the reason I like to talk about the initials study on the first day of class is that the researchers used a particularly convincing measure of ill health: being dead. It's not a perfect measure, because there are plenty of people who die from an unfortunate accident but were otherwise in fine health. But in general, people who live a long time are healthier than people who do not. Plus, it is rather unlikely that death will be measured incorrectly, whereas if, for example, you have to ask people how many sick days they took last year, it is easy for them to make a mistake. In the study of initials, men with positive initials lived an average of seven years longer than men with negative initials. That's a giant effect, and I find it quite interesting, but the only reason anyone takes this odd finding at all seriously is that death is a convincing measure of health. Anything less persuasive and my students might have tried to deny that there was a relationship between initials and health. But it's hard to deny death.

I told you that long story partly to explain why I think the most important evidence regarding whether obesity causes poor health comes from studies of life and death. If obesity really is unhealthy, obese people should have shorter life spans than thinner people. Do they? This seemingly simple question has been addressed in more than a hundred studies, which, combined, included millions of participants. All of that information was compiled in one tour de force article[7] by a biostatistician name Katherine Flegal.

From each study, Flegal first calculated the risk of death (during a certain period of time) for people who were categorized as normal weight (BMI of 18.5–25) and overweight (BMI of 25–30). Then she calculated the ratio of the death rates for overweight people compared to normal-weight people.[8] If the risk of death for overweight people is the same as the risk of death for normal-weight people, then this ratio will equal 1. If the risk of death for overweight people is higher than for normal-weight people, the risk ratio will be larger than 1. The more deadly being overweight is, the larger this number should be.

Although it is a highly technical paper, the results are perfectly clear. In 93 percent of the studies, the risk ratios equaled 1, showing that overweight people were at least as healthy as normal-weight people.[9] In fact, combining the data from all 140 studies, Flegal found that overweight people had a slightly lower risk of death than normal-weight people. Being overweight appears to be even a bit healthier than being the recommended weight.

Then Flegal repeated the whole process for people who were categorized as obesity class I (BMIs from 30 to 35). In 87 percent of the studies, the risk ratios again equaled 1, showing that people in this weight category (which is the majority of obese people) were just as healthy as normal-weight people. Only when Flegal looked at people in obesity class II (BMI of 35–40) and higher (BMI>40; what you might have heard referred to as "morbid obesity") did she find risk ratios larger than 1. Even then, the majority of the studies (64 percent) had ratios equal to 1. So in two out of three studies, even the very heaviest obese individuals had the same risk of death as normal-weight people. In fact, the only group of people who had a higher overall risk of death than normal-weight people were people in obesity class II and up who were also under the age of 65. For those people, their ratio of risk compared to normal-weight people was 1.3. To help put that number in perspective, the ratio of risk for lung cancer[10] among smokers compared to nonsmokers is over 30. In the handful of articles that separates obesity class II from obesity classes III and up, it is clear that it is obesity class III and up, not class II, that is the culprit here. Only 6 percent of the U.S. population has a BMI that high.[11]

Being overweight or obese (at least classes I and II) is not going to kill you, but interestingly, being underweight (BMI<18.5) may be a problem. Although Flegal didn't include underweight people in her tour de force article, she did include it in an earlier paper. She found that people categorized as underweight had a higher risk of death than normal-weight people.[12] This was even true when she did special analyses to control for smoking status and to rule out the possibility that people were underweight because they had serious diseases that caused them to lose weight. We are told that skinny is healthy, but it just might not be.

THE OBESITY PARADOX

The mortality evidence is important because mortality is the most straightforward and convincing measure of health. But there is more to life than not being dead, so it's also important to consider whether obese people suffer from more diseases or have a worse quality of life than thinner people.

Here again, the findings are not what you might expect. Overweight and obese people are more likely than normal-weight people to be diagnosed with several diseases, particularly diabetes, and cardiovascular diseases.[13] These are serious diseases that cause a lot of suffering, and their link to obesity is undeniable. But it's not a perfect link. You would think that rates of these diseases would have skyrocketed over the decades in which obesity rates more than doubled, but they didn't. The prevalence of diabetes went from 9 percent to 11 percent,[14] and rates of cardiovascular diseases, which are supposed to be the most serious and alarming consequence of obesity, actually decreased from 12 percent to 11 percent.[15]

Not only that, but once people have a disease, overweight and obese people may even have a better prognosis than normal-weight people. This has been shown for cardiovascular diseases (hypertension, heart failure, coronary heart disease),[16] stroke,[17] diabetes,[18] kidney disease,[19] chronic obstructive lung disease,[20] rheumatoid arthritis,[21] pneumonia,[22] and even advanced lung[23] and prostate[24] cancer. This pattern is found so often that it has a name: the obesity paradox.

This obesity paradox is surprising to the masses of people who have never thought to question the relationship between obesity and health. So far, researchers cannot explain why this happens. Some researchers have suggested that overweight and obese people may be protected from malnutrition when they have illnesses that cause significant weight loss, as in many cancers and AIDS.[25] They have also suggested that specific hormonal patterns that occur in obesity may be protective.[26] But this paradox remains unsolved, for now.

IS IT REALLY THE CULPRIT?

Even if people who are very obese are more likely to die or develop certain illnesses than non-obese people, it still does not mean that their weight is the *cause* of those problems. To be fair, the same goes for the studies showing that obesity leads to better prognoses once people have certain diseases. Those studies do not show that obesity causes better prognoses. In fact, there are no studies that show that obesity causes health problems, and no studies that show obesity causes health benefits. The important word here is "causes." Showing that obesity is the cause of a health problem (or health benefit) is a difficult scientific problem.

Showing that one thing causes another requires a randomized controlled trial, which, as we discussed in Chapter 1, is the gold standard of scientific study design. Without randomly assigning people to be obese or not, researchers cannot draw conclusions about what obesity does or does not cause.[27] Of course, this kind of obesity study does not exist—at least not with people. It would be unethical, as well as flat-out ridiculous. Imagine signing up to be a participant in a study. You figure you can aid science and also earn a little money for your efforts. The researcher approaches you with a coin. He says that he will flip it, and that if it comes up heads, you will have to gain enough weight to become obese (if you aren't already obese), and then stay obese for, well, ever, so that he can see what diseases you get and how long you live. If it comes up tails, you will have to become normal-weight (if you aren't already), and then stay at that weight forever. Not only is this unethical, it's not even possible.

It's not possible because, as we've discussed, people can't easily gain enough weight to become obese and stay that way (or lose enough weight to become thin and stay that way). If people assigned to become obese did become obese, but then lost the weight, they would no longer be a useful test of the health effects of being obese. In addition to that, remember that a thin person who purposely gains weight is different, biologically, from a person who was obese for most of his or her life. So anything researchers learn from thin people who are assigned to get fat (or fat people who are assigned to get thin)—even if people can maintain their assigned weight for long enough—may not apply to people who have always been thin or fat.[28]

Another possibility, then, is to do the opposite kind of study: take obese people, randomly assign them to become thin or not, and then track them over the next several decades. If obesity is bad for you, then surely becoming thin would be good for you, right? The closest thing we have to studies like this are long-term diet studies[29] like those we looked at in Chapter 1. In those studies, participants were randomly assigned to diet or to not diet, and then they were studied for two or more years after that. Of course, participants didn't generally become thin, and the majority of them regained most of the weight they lost, so researchers can't say much about whether there are health benefits from no longer being obese. But still, if obesity is unhealthy, then the more weight people manage to keep off, the healthier they should get.

To see if we could find evidence that losing weight improves health, Janet Tomiyama, Britt Ahlstrom, and I dug back into each of those long-term diet studies to see if they included any measures of health. None of the studies measured death, very few measured whether people developed diseases, but many measured blood pressure, cholesterol, triglyceride, and blood glucose levels. We looked at whether those measures of health improved, when people kept the weight off. They did not. The participants' health, at least according to those outcomes, was unrelated to their weight loss.[30]

There is one study[31] that is often cited because its participants did manage to keep off a substantial amount of weight for a long period of time. It was designed to look at the long-term effects of weight loss in overweight and obese people with type 2 diabetes, and it was a highly respected and methodologically rigorous study. Nearly ten years after the study began, participants had kept off 6 percent of their starting weight. This may not seem like a lot of weight—if you started off at 200 pounds, 6 percent would be about 12 pounds—but since the government has defined "successful dieting" as keeping off 5 percent of your starting weight, this was considered to be impressive.

The health benefits from this weight loss, however, were not impressive, even to the government. The National Institutes of Health ended the fifteen-year, $15 million study two years ahead of schedule for the official reason of "futility," which means that they could already conclude that there was a "low likelihood of finding a benefit of the intervention."[32] In this case, statisticians determined that given the minimal health benefits they'd observed so far, it would be nearly impossible to show over the next two years that the diet was actually helping to prevent strokes, heart attacks, or deaths from cardiovascular disease, which is what the diet was designed to prevent.[33] There were other benefits to the diet program though. Most important, diet participants were better able to manage their diabetes without medication than control participants.[34] That's a good thing, but it wasn't good enough for the government to keep funding the study.

OTHER DIFFERENCES BETWEEN OBESE AND NON-OBESE PEOPLE

Most studies on obesity and health[35] compare people who are already obese to people who are already non-obese, instead of randomly assigning people to be obese or not.[36] This is a problem, scientifically speaking, because already obese people are not only different from non-obese people in terms of their weight, but they are different in lots of other ways, too. For example, obese people are less likely to exercise than non-obese people,[37] so if they get sick more often, there is no way to know from this kind of study if they got sick because they weigh more, or because they exercise less. The automatic assumption of most people is that obesity is the culprit, but there is reason to believe that other factors matter just as much, or even more. Let's look closely at some of the pre-existing differences between obese and non-obese people to see if they might account for health problems that we typically blame on obesity.

Differences in Level of Physical Fitness

Obese people are more likely to be sedentary than non-obese people,[38] and we all know that being sedentary is bad for us and that exercising is good for us.[39] Unlike studying the overall impact of obesity on health, which is not possible, it is possible to study the effects of exercise. Researchers can randomly assign some participants to exercise and some to be sedentary, and then determine if the exercise is beneficial to the participants' health, maybe not for a very long period of time, but for quite a while. There are even studies that require participants to exercise in front of researchers so that researchers can be sure the participants really did it.[40]

We know from these studies that exercise benefits your health in many ways, including reducing risk factors for type 2 diabetes[41] and improving blood sugar control among people with diabetes.[42] It has also been found to reduce mortality among patients with coronary heart disease[43] as well as to prevent cardiovascular disease,[44] raise high-density lipoprotein ("good") cholesterol, lower triglycerides, and decrease blood pressure in people with hypertension.[45] There is also suggestive evidence that exercise may protect against colon cancer[46] and breast cancer,[47] although these cancer findings were not from studies that could test causality.

We can't know for sure what role exercise plays in the health profiles of obese and non-obese people, but we do know that exercise has been shown to improve your health even when it doesn't lead to weight loss.[48] Active obese individuals have lower rates of sickness and mortality than non-obese sedentary people.[49] In one study of older men, for example, the obese men who were physically fit had lower mortality rates than men of all sizes who were not physically fit.[50] Since the health benefits of exercise do not require you to be thin, it seems plausible that your health has more to do with your fitness level than with your weight.

Differences in Weight Cycling

We know that weight cycling—yo-yo dieting—may cause all sorts of health problems. And who is likely to have weight cycled the most? Obese people.[51] If weight cycling causes health problems, and if obese people are more likely than non-obese people to have weight cycled, then any differences in health between obese and non-obese people could be at least partially attributed to weight cycling, rather than the excess weight itself.

Differences in Socioeconomic Status

There are enormous differences between people in this country in wealth, status, and education. The sum of these three factors is called socioeconomic status, or SES, and it is strongly correlated with health.[52] People with low SES have worse health—no matter how you measure health—than people with high SES.

They have shorter life spans[53] and are more likely to have diseases such as cardiovascular disease, diabetes, hypertension, metabolic syndrome, arthritis, and respiratory disease.[54] The relationship between SES and health is so strong that addressing it (and other health inequities) was listed as one of the four overarching goals in the ten-year health agenda the U.S. government published in 2010.[55]

There are many reasons why people with low SES are more likely to become ill than people with higher SES,[56] including reduced access to good quality health care (or perhaps any health care at all). People with low SES tend to lead more stressful lives, with concerns about job security and financial obligations, as well as access to proper shelter and sufficient healthy food. The daily stresses can add up, leading to health problems across many systems of the body.[57] People with low SES also have more dangerous jobs, live in more dangerous neighborhoods, and are more likely to be exposed to environmental toxins and carcinogens than people with higher SES.[58]

Importantly, obese people have lower SES than non-obese people,[59] and these differences may partially account for health differences between them. It's not hard to imagine. People with low SES may gain weight because they can only afford to eat junk food and may not have time or a safe place to exercise. They may also gain weight because of the increased amount of stress they experience. Gaining weight, in turn, could make it hard for them to find a job due to weight-based discrimination. This could further lower their SES, which could then lead to worse health. In sum, obesity and low SES may form a vicious cycle in which low SES makes obesity more likely and discrimination due to obesity lowers people's SES. At least some of the relationship between obesity and health is likely accounted for by differences in SES.[60]

Differences in the Distribution of Fat on Your Body

You may have noticed an unfamiliar disease—metabolic syndrome—on the list of diseases that people with low SES are more likely to develop. Metabolic syndrome is not actually a disease, rather, it is a cluster of symptoms that tend to occur together and indicate that a person is at risk for cardiovascular disease and diabetes. People are diagnosed with metabolic syndrome if they have at least three of these five symptoms: high blood pressure, high fasting blood sugar, high triglyceride level, low HDL (good) cholesterol, and high waist circumference.[61]

Your waist circumference is a useful indication of your body composition, or how fat happens to be distributed on your body. If you have a high waist circumference, your body will likely have the apple shape: bigger belly, smaller legs. This generally means that you have increased visceral fat, which is the kind of fat that gets packed around the organs in your abdomen, and which is linked to health problems. If your waist circumference is on the lower side, your body will likely have the pear shape, with more fat distributed on your hips and thighs than in your belly. This kind of fat, called subcutaneous fat, is not related to health problems.

Waist circumference is of course related to obesity, but it is also importantly different from it. There are many obese people with a relatively low waist circumference, as well as non-obese people with a high waist circumference (imagine a skinny guy with a beer belly). Studies have carefully teased out the effects of your weight and your waist circumference on health, and they show that waist circumference is what matters. A higher waist circumference leads to a higher risk of mortality, regardless of your weight.[62] In fact, the people with the highest risk of mortality in one study were people who were at a "healthy" weight, but who had a high waist circumference. People who were obese but had a low waist circumference had the lowest death rate.[63]

So what matters is how your weight is distributed on your body, rather than how much weight there is, and it is the apple pattern that is problematic, not the pear pattern. Think about the people in your life who are apple-shaped. Notice anything they have in common? Odds are, they are mainly men. And odds are, most pear-shaped people you know are women. I can't think of any pear-shaped men that I know. And I can only bring to mind one apple-shaped woman. Even if women are obese, since they generally carry their excess weight in their hips and thighs, they have less to worry about than men with the same amount of excess weight, but carried in the belly.

Differences in Medical Care

For many people, the hardest thing about being obese is enduring the stigma and discrimination that accompany it. In our increasingly open-minded culture, most people wouldn't discriminate (or at least admit to discriminating) against others based on their gender or ethnic group, but people are still willing to admit that they discriminate against obese people. The more discrimination people experience, the worse their health.[64] In effect, weight stigma can make you ill.[65]

One way that this discrimination can lead to illness is when it keeps people from accessing good quality medical care. If you avoid going to the doctor, you are less likely to benefit from early intervention and treatment of preventable diseases. Obese people often say that they avoid the medical system because they feel they are treated disrespectfully by doctors,[66] that doctors make inappropriate comments about their weight,[67] and that they are given unsolicited weight loss advice[68] when seeking treatment unrelated to weight loss (such as for an ear infection or a broken toe).

Unfortunately, it is not the case that obese people are being paranoid or are misperceiving doctors' attitudes toward them. I wish they were. Doctors freely admit these attitudes. On one survey of more than 600 physicians, at least half reported viewing obese patients as awkward, unattractive, and noncompliant, and a third rated them as weak-willed, sloppy, and lazy.[69] At a scientific convention on the study and treatment of obesity, fat people were rated as more lazy, stupid, and worthless than thin people by obesity researchers and doctors who care for obese patients.[70] If you specialize in obesity, shouldn't you be more understanding than this?

These negative views translate into worse care. In another study, doctors were asked to give their treatment plan for a patient based on her medical chart. They were given one of several medical charts that (unbeknownst to them) were created to be identical except for the patient's weight.[71] The doctors reported less desire to help the obese patients, said that seeing them would feel more like a waste of their time, and said that they would spend less time with them. Audio recordings of outpatient visits show that doctors were less empathic and warm with obese patients than non-obese patients.[72] Medical students—our future doctors—also show strong biases against obese people.[73]

Given these biases, it is not surprising that obese people are 50 percent more likely than non-obese people to have changed doctors five or more times.[74] Switching doctors disrupts the continuity of care, prevents the development of a strong doctor-patient relationship, and leaves patients with periods of time in which they don't have a primary care doctor, increasing their likelihood of needing to seek treatment in the emergency room. Even more alarming, obese people are less likely than non-obese people to be screened for cervical cancer,[75] breast cancer,[76] and colorectal cancer,[77] and they are less likely to have gotten a flu vaccine.[78]

Differences in Stress

Weight stigma can also make you sick by causing stress, leading to all of the many health problems that stress brings about. Dozens of studies show that being stigmatized based on race, gender, or other traits is linked to stress.[79] Many of these studies are able to show that stigma isn't just associated with stress, but that stigma causes stress. They can show the causal connection because in those studies, researchers randomly assigned participants to experience discrimination or not, right there in a lab. That sounds a little harsh, I know, but they keep it brief and mild and when the experiment ends clearly explain what they were up to. They might have participants write an essay, for example, and then give them sexist feedback on it. In other studies they ask people to think about events from their past in which they experienced discrimination.

In one particularly clever study, obese and non-obese women had to prepare and then give a speech about why they would be a good person to date.[80] Half of the women were instructed to give their speech on camera. The rest were audiotaped as they gave their speech. It sounds a bit horrifying either way, but for the women speaking on camera, concerns about how viewers would react to their weight would be heightened, whereas the women who were audiotaped did not have to worry about that. Sure enough, for the women who were videotaped, the more they weighed, the more their blood pressure increased while they gave their speech. This did not happen to the audiotaped women. Notice that the women did not experience any discrimination during the study, but in the videotape condition they knew there was the possibility that it could happen later.

The fact that relatively minor episodes of discrimination in the lab, reminders of past discrimination, or the possibility of future discrimination cause a physiological stress response is both remarkable and troubling. It is remarkable that subtle psychological experiences have physiological effects (though not surprising to health psychologists), and troubling because outside of the lab, obese people experience larger and more consequential forms of discrimination, and for many obese people, it happens relentlessly.[81]

THE BOTTOM LINE

We are often warned about the health effects of becoming overweight or obese. And there are many noted health differences between obese and non-obese people. But there are also a multitude of ways in which obese and non-obese people differ from one another beyond simply how much they weigh. These differences are not a secret to obesity researchers, and yet they continue to report studies comparing the health of obese people to non-obese people, blame obesity for causing the health problems of obese people, and rarely acknowledge the potential of alternative explanations.

But variables such as exercise, weight cycling, socioeconomic status, fat distribution, and discrimination all factor into a person's overall health. And there are many other factors that may also be significant. Obese people eat more unhealthy trans fats and less healthy fiber, fruits, and vegetables than do non-obese people, and these nutrition differences may influence their health.[82] Obese people consume more artificial sweeteners (for example, in diet soda),[83] and these sweeteners have been linked to increased levels of cardiovascular disease,[84] as well as glucose intolerance, which can lead to diabetes.[85] Obese people are also more likely to use diet drugs,[86] and over the years, many of these drugs have been found to be dangerous, causing hypertension, valvular heart disease, or other cardiovascular problems.[87] In addition, obese people are more likely to be lonely or socially isolated,[88] and loneliness has been found to be associated with mortality.[89]

There are statistical techniques that can be used to minimize the extent to which these kinds of variables bias study results. They are routinely used to account for age and gender differences, but it is not routine to use them for these other potential forms of bias. I went through the list of ninety-seven studies on obesity and mortality that Katherine Flegal included in her thorough review and counted how many studies controlled for each of these factors.[90] Physical activity was the most likely to be statistically controlled for, but that was done in fewer than half of the studies. Only sixteen of the studies took socioeconomic status into account,[91] one study controlled for distribution of body fat, and none accounted for weight cycling, stigma or stress, or use of diet drugs. No study controlled for more than two of these factors, and half didn't control for any. When researchers fail to statistically control for these factors in their studies on obesity and health, they make obesity look more dangerous than it is.

Even with all of the statistical flaws in obesity studies, the actual difference in life expectancy that they find between people who are obese (class I) and people who are normal weight is one year.[92] And that difference goes away for people age sixty-five or over.[93] You know what that means? Your life expectancy is about six years shorter if you have the initials F.A.T.[94] than if you *are* fat (class I obese).

Why has the case that obesity will kill you been overstated? Partly it's because the media tends to overhype health headlines.[95] Partly it's because the medical community fears that if people don't think obesity is a death trap, they'll stop trying to eat a healthy diet and end up behaving in truly unhealthy ways. But you also have to look at which scientists are saying that obesity will kill you: Scientists with a vested interest in that being true. Scientists who are taking money from companies that sell diet drugs and other weight loss products. Scientists who sit on the boards of directors of these companies. Researchers are required to list these conflicts of interest at the end of articles they publish in medical journals,[96] and in obesity research, you could use these lists as a handy directory of companies in the weight loss industry.

Think I'm exaggerating? Consider the scientists who claimed that the current generation of children would have a shorter life expectancy than their parents,[97] which isn't close to true (and which they don't even seem to believe themselves).[98] The conflict of interest statement at the end of that paper says that one of the authors received "grants, monetary donations, donations of product, payments for consultation, contracts, honoraria or commitments thereof" from 148 companies, most of which are weight loss and pharmaceutical companies.[99] Those companies include Weight Watchers, Jenny Craig, and Slim-Fast; the makers of weight loss drugs Xenical, Meridia, and Redux; plus four companies that produced the dangerous combination diet drug fen-phen, along with the law firm that defended those companies in court. As a comparison, the biostatistician who summarized all the mortality studies and found that obesity was probably not going to kill you did not receive money from any companies at all.[100]

I hope you're not still under the impression that you have to diet or else obesity will kill you. If you exercise, eat nutritiously, avoid weight cycling, and get good quality medical care, you don't need to worry about obesity shortening your life. Especially if you shield yourself from weight stigma and the stress it causes, which we'll talk about in Part IV. But now let's talk about smart regulation strategies for living at the lower end of your set weight range. These strategies will painlessly stabilize your eating and keep your weight from yo-yoing.

PART THREE

HOW TO REACH YOUR LEANEST LIVABLE WEIGHT

(NO WILLPOWER REQUIRED)

. . . .

CHAPTER 6

LESSONS FROM A LEAN PIG

One day I got a phone call from a stranger who told me that he had lost a lot of weight on a diet and wanted to know if he was doomed to regain it. Believe it or not, I get lots of calls like this. Since I don't know these people or their individual circumstances, I tend to respond by saying that yes, the majority of people who lose weight on a diet will gain it back at some point, but that there is a small minority who successfully keep it off. I can't predict what will happen to any particular person. Usually, the conversation ends there. But this time, I stayed on the phone. The voice on the other end, Mac Nelson,[1] was a seventy-four-year-old man from rural Texas with a thick accent. He said that he had figured out the secret to keeping weight off. From his pig. Since pigs are not known for their svelte figures, I was intrigued.

He told me that when he was young, he raised a pig for the state fair. His friends did, too, and the pigs all came from the same litter. His friends fed their pigs the standard way: They left the food in a self-feeder in the pigs' pen, so the pigs had access to it all day long and could eat whenever they wanted. Mac didn't have a self-feeder for his pig, and even though his Future Farmers of America instructor told him to build one, he never got around to it. Instead, he brought out a slop bucket twice a day, and let the pig eat as much as it wanted.

When it was time to bring the pigs to the state fair for judging, Mac's pig had grown to be strong, healthy, and lean, while his friends' pigs had grown strong, healthy, and fat. Fatness is prized in pigs, so Mac's pig "got beat," as he put it. But Mac had an insight about eating that he remembered and made use of years later, when he wanted to lose weight. He realized that the longer there was food in front of him, the more he would eat. So he began eating twice a day—whatever he wanted, as much as he wanted. But that was it; he didn't eat anything else all day. Over the years, he weighed himself once a month and wrote down the number on the scale (he sent me a photograph of the piece of paper that held the tally). Mac lost 42 pounds in two years, and has kept it off for seven years and counting.

I'm not endorsing the Mac Nelson diet plan, because eating only twice a day sounds miserable (though it wasn't for Mac), but his main insight is right on the money and is the basis for the three strategies for weight management that I'll share in this chapter: If it's not there, you can't eat it, and if it is there, you will. These are smart regulation strategies, because they rely on our brains rather than the brute strength of our limited willpower to resist temptation.

Pioneering self-control researcher Walter Mischel noted that the way kids in his classic marshmallow self-control studies managed to resist eating the marshmallow was by "converting the difficult conflict from one requiring acts of self-denial and grim determination to a more playful enjoyable time."[2] Instead of staring at the marshmallow, they covered their eyes, turned their back, pretended the marshmallow was a cloud, sang songs, or played games with their hands or feet. They succeeded at self-control by changing the situation so that self-control was not needed. This is smart regulation, and you are going to use it to reach and stay at your leanest livable weight.

SMART REGULATION STRATEGY 1: ENCOUNTER
LESS TEMPTATION BY CREATING OBSTACLES

There are two different routes that I can take to the office each day. One route involves a freeway that is slow and crowded during rush hour, but speedy the rest of the time. The other involves surface streets that have a lot of annoying traffic lights, but the route is faster than the freeway during rush hour. Because of this, I generally choose my route based on the time of day. When I want a treat, however, no matter what time of day it is, I choose the surface streets. On that route, I pass my favorite bakery. My resistance to that bakery is nonexistent. Some mornings I wrestle with this decision, and frequently I lose the battle and take the bakery route. But if I am trying to limit my calorie intake, I take the freeway, regardless of what time of day it is.

There are many aspects of your day that might benefit from this strategy.[3] Where do you encounter tempting foods? How about lunchtime at work? Do you tend to go out for lunch? Most of the time you will eat a healthier, lower-calorie meal if you bring it yourself, rather than eating in a restaurant. I have a handy obstacle to going out: winter. Specifically, Minnesota winter. I can't bear to go out in the cold when it's nonessential, so in the winter, it is easy for me to avoid going out to lunch. During the other five months of the year, I arrange my day so that I am unable to go out to lunch. I schedule my meetings so that I don't have enough time between them to go out to eat. That keeps me stuck in the office, so I need to rely on whatever I have packed for myself. Another obstacle at work is that despite your careful planning, your colleagues can sabotage your best efforts—a coworker brings in a box of doughnuts on a Friday morning, or there's a party in the conference room to celebrate someone's birthday with a few dozen cupcakes. In my lab, there is near-constant temptation from leftover food hanging around from our eating studies. It's hard to resist these items when they're right in front of you, but you can make an effort to avoid encountering them by staying out of the office kitchen or skipping out on the birthday party. In my case, I try to stay in my office rather than going into the lab, where the food is kept.

Sometimes the temptation is already right there on your dinner plate, and there is nothing harder to resist than food on your own plate. In fact, in recorded history, there are no documented instances of this occurring. Okay, I made that up, but still, this is the last thing you want to have to do. It's not just difficult, but it feels bad—it makes you feel deprived if you can't eat it, or guilty if you throw it away. When you prepare your own food, don't put yourself in a situation where you have to resist some of the food that is on your plate—only serve yourself a reasonable portion that you can feel good about eating.

When we eat out, we have a lot less control over what's on our plate—and as we all know, restaurant serving sizes are completely out of control. Serving sizes of convenience foods and drinks are, too.[4] Think about the size of the drinks we buy. The bottle that Coca-Cola patented in 1916 held 6.5 ounces of soda. Now it is not uncommon to buy Coke in a cup that holds a quart (32 ounces) or half gallon (64 ounces) of soda. Newer models of cars even come with larger cup holders to accommodate these massive containers.[5]

In high school I worked part-time at a Baskin-Robbins ice cream store. In 1983, when I first started, my boss taught me the mantra, "Think 2.5 ounces," because that was the size a scoop of ice cream was supposed to be. He had me weigh every scoop until I got accustomed to what 2.5 ounces looked and felt like. A couple of years later, while I was still working there, the company introduced the 4-ounce scoop. A scoop that large was so unusual, the company had to have larger ice cream scoopers specially made.[6] Four ounces is now the standard size for ice cream scoops at most national ice cream chains, and 2.5 ounces is considered a child-size scoop, if it's offered at all. Similarly, McDonald's french fries originally came in only one portion size, and that size is now considered the small.[7] Newer editions of *The Joy of Cooking* have the same cookie recipes as the original edition, but these same quantities of butter, flour, and sugar are now described as making fewer—but larger— cookies.[8] One serving is not what it used to be.

My favorite piece of evidence about the increase in portion sizes comes from a study comparing the size of the foods in different paintings of the Last Supper from over the centuries.[9] To control for the different-sized paintings, the researchers did their comparisons by calculating a food-to-head ratio. Presumably heads have not gotten larger in that time. Over the years, however, the bread, entrees, and plates all did.[10]

There is plenty of evidence that the larger the portion, the more you eat.[11] The larger the cereal box (or any box) you serve yourself from, the more you take and the more you eat.[12] The larger the serving spoon you serve yourself with or the serving bowl you serve yourself from, the more you take and the more you eat.[13] You'll even eat more from one big chocolate bar than you would if you were given that same amount of chocolate, but in several small bars.[14]

You can easily change the portion sizes in your own home. I wouldn't suggest this if it would feel like deprivation, but there is plenty of research showing that for most people, it doesn't. This comforting evidence comes courtesy of Brian Wansink, head of Cornell's Food & Brand Lab and author of *Mindless Eating*. In one of his clever food studies he created a bottomless soup bowl: a bowl that subtly refills itself while you eat from it, so it never looks like it is emptying.[15] How'd he do that? Something complicated with tubes and pipes and pressure physics. But what he learned by having study participants unknowingly eat from this deceptive bowl is that people have no idea how much they are eating, and they decide how full they feel based on what they see, not how they feel. So if they see that their bowl of soup is full, they assume they haven't eaten much, and that they are still hungry, even though they may have eaten the equivalent of two (or more) full bowls.[16]

But we can also take advantage of this concept in reverse. If you use a smaller plate and fill it up, you think you are eating more food, because food on a small plate looks like more food than that same amount of food on a big plate.[17] This tricks you into feeling full sooner, and amazingly, it still works even when you know about it.[18] The small plate also forces you to serve yourself less food, and the less you have on your plate, the less you eat.[19] There's no need to rely on willpower to resist anything.

There is one recent phenomenon working against the portion size trend. Even though standard portion sizes are larger than they used to be, some foods are starting to come in slightly smaller packages than before. Companies are sneakily trying to hide price increases by putting less food in the package, but keeping the price the same. This is presumably more tolerable to consumers than price increases, but no consumer I know has been anything but annoyed when they noticed this subterfuge. One ice cream brand now has only 14 ounces of ice cream in what it absurdly continues to call its pint, but the price is the same as it was when it had 16 ounces in it, and the package looks the same.[20] If this continues, corporate greed may lead people to eat less without realizing it.

No Obstacle Is Too Small

Want to know a secret to saving money on toilet paper? Just squish the roll a bit (to make it flatter) before putting it on its spindle. It won't turn as easily, so it will be incrementally harder to rip toilet paper off the roll. When that happens, people use less. This is a tiny inconvenience. I might even argue that this is the tiniest possible inconvenience. And yet it alters people's behavior enough that this tip routinely turns up as a suggestion for thriftiness in blogs about saving money.[21]

Here's why it works: People are lazy. Even the most hardworking among us are, on some level, pretty lazy. At the very least, we are constantly assessing situations for the path of least resistance—or, to put it another way, the path with the fewest obstacles.

Another, more serious example of the effectiveness of tiny obstacles was documented in the United Kingdom, after laws required acetaminophen (Tylenol) to be packaged in small blister packs instead of bottles.[22] To use the medication from a blister pack, each individual pill must be pushed out of the packaging separately from the other pills, and it is harder to grab a handful at once. That small obstacle to accessing pills was linked to a 21 percent reduction in suicides and accidental poisonings from the over-the-counter drug.

I am not suggesting that potato chips should be packaged in individual blister packs. But how snack food is packaged and presented, and where it is located, can make a big difference in whether or not you eat it. Researchers at Utrecht University did a study in which they measured how much candy people ate in relation to the proximity of the candy dish.[23] The researchers found that people ate less candy when the dish was across the room from them than when the dish was right next to them. Walking less than five feet across a room should not be an effective obstacle, but it was. Perhaps that part doesn't surprise you. Getting up from your chair and walking across the room is a real obstacle—it causes you to take a pause in your work, get up, and walk around. But it turns out that the candy doesn't even need to be that far away. Merely having to extend your arm across a table was shown to be as much of a deterrent as having to walk across the room. Why? Because people are lazy, so tiny obstacles can be formidable. You might be thinking that if you did go to all the trouble of walking across the room to get some candy, you would probably make it worth your while and take a lot. That feels to me like what I would do. The researchers wondered about that, too, so they looked at the behavior of just the people who did walk over to the dish. Those people did not take or eat more candy than the people who took candy from the closer dishes.[24] So being farther away did not have a downside.

Laziness leads to less eating in other situations, too. At salad bars, people eat less of the foods that they have to reach the slightest bit farther under the sneeze shields to get. They also eat less of foods served with tongs, which require a little more effort to operate than a spoon.[25] Similarly, if you are not particularly adept at eating with chopsticks, you will likely eat less when you use them compared to when you use a fork.[26]

In 2012, the city of New York passed a law banning restaurants, movie theaters, and sports stadiums from selling drinks in cups larger than sixteen ounces, with the goal of reducing soda consumption. The ban spawned thousands of jokes and critiques, many pointing out that people still could drink as much soda as they wanted by purchasing multiple cups, and that all the law would do was inconvenience them.[27] The inconvenience, however, is exactly why I thought the ban was a good idea, and indeed, it was the point of the ban. Having to get back in line to purchase another beverage is a much larger obstacle than, say, reaching out your arm, serving yourself tomato slices with tongs, or rotating a slightly smushed toilet paper roll. Alas, to the disappointment of public health officials, as well as to data geeks like myself, the law was overturned and we'll never know what would have happened.

But effort isn't the only effective obstacle in preventing over-eating. Other obstacles are effective because they make the food less noticeable or distract you from it. For example, in an effort to get employees to stop eating so much of the free candy that is readily available at Google's New York office, M&Ms were switched from clear containers to opaque ones. In the first seven weeks after this change, the 2,000 employees ate 3 million fewer calories from M&Ms than they had eaten in the seven weeks before the change.[28]

I've seen every member in my family use this strategy without even knowing they're doing it. My kids use it in restaurants to resist drinking their entire soda before the meal is served. We don't let them have soda very often, so this is difficult. They manage it by pushing their cups out of their line of sight and as far away from themselves as possible until the entrees arrive. Similarly, one evening in a Mexican restaurant I realized that my husband had moved the basket of tortilla chips entirely off our table and onto the windowsill to stop himself from eating them.

I take advantage of the small obstacle strategy, too, when I make a pan of Rice Krispies treats, which are pretty close to irresistible to me. There is no place in my house that is far enough away for distance to be a sufficient obstacle on its own. If I leave the pan on the counter, I go back and forth, cutting myself thin slice after thin slice, until it is mostly gone. But I find that if I cut myself a decent-sized slab, put the knife in the dishwasher, cover the pan with tin foil, and put it in the fridge, I end up eating much less than if the pan were left uncovered on the counter. The knife part is important. If I leave the knife in the pan with the Rice Krispies treats, it is too easy to cut another little slice off. But the knife in the dishwasher is another small barrier. Not only do I have to go to the effort of getting another knife, but I also have to convince myself that it is worth it to dirty another knife for this purpose. And seeing the pileup of knives also becomes an embarrassing deterrent, reminding me of how much I have been eating. The beauty of these strategies is that they help you eat a little less, but without suffering for it. When I cut myself a piece, I end up feeling like I ate a lot, since I can see the whole piece at once. Those thin slices add up to more than the one piece, but it doesn't look like it at the time, and it doesn't feel like it.

SMART REGULATION STRATEGY 2: MAKE HEALTHY FOODS MORE ACCESSIBLE AND NOTICEABLE

Creating small obstacles can help us limit how much unhealthy food we eat, but when we want to eat *more* of a certain kind of food, we want to do the opposite: remove as many barriers as possible. For example, if you want to eat more fruits and vegetables, make them easier to access. Make them unavoidable. Have a fruit bowl (with fruit in it) on your table. Sounds obvious and too easy, doesn't it? But it works.[29] Having the fruit in ready-to-eat form helps, too. The effort of peeling an orange can be an insurmountable obstacle, no matter how good a peeler you are. Peeling bananas, on the other hand, is a no-brainer, so they are easily eaten from a fruit bowl. Grapes are even easier, because all you have to do is grab some. At dinner on campus at the University of Cambridge, I was surprised to see that the fruit bowl on the table didn't just sit there like a table centerpiece, but it got passed around from person to person. Much more fruit was eaten because of it. And not surprisingly, the smaller, more bite-sized fruits were the first ones taken. People took handfuls of grapes, dates, and adorable tiny bananas.

Fruit is easy compared to vegetables. Vegetables have a lot of obstacles to overcome, including not being as sweet as fruits. But an even bigger problem is that many of them are high maintenance. They need to be cleaned well, parts of them need to be cut off, some need to be peeled, and many require some degree of cooking or seasoning to be appealing. These are big barriers to eating vegetables, even once you've bought them and they are safely in your house. This is why you need to at least partially prepare your vegetables the moment you get them home from the store.

Prepping your vegetables ahead of time can be a pain, but it's worth it.[30] We get a weekly farm share during the summer and fall (and once, regrettably, during a Minnesota season referred to as "deep winter"). The day we pick up the multiple bags of vegetables, my husband washes and trims everything, and chops the vegetables into usable-size pieces. He roasts beets, rutabaga, celeriac, and turnips, which is the only hope those vegetables have of being eaten, at least in our house. We manage to eat our entire farm share each week (even in deep winter), and I am convinced it is because he invests time breaking down the obstacles that would otherwise keep us from eating our vegetables.

Everyone's barriers are different, so spend some time thinking about the things that consistently prevent you from eating healthy food, and then come up with creative ways to knock those barriers down. For example, if you never have healthy food in the house because you don't have time to get to the grocery store, try shopping online and have your produce delivered. Does it take you forever to chop your vegetables? Buy them prechopped. Want to add legumes to your diet but never remember to soak them overnight? Use canned beans. Need to feed your family the moment you get home from work? Try using a slow cooker once a week. I turn it on before work and dinner is ready and waiting when I get home.

SMART REGULATION STRATEGY 3: BE ALONE WITH A VEGETABLE

I've left my favorite vegetable-eating strategy for last. The idea for this strategy comes from something I witnessed my children do as we sat in a deli in Los Angeles (they were about three and six years old). Typically, the waitress puts down a nice bowl of pickles on the table when you arrive, but this particular day they must have run out of pickles, so they brought us a large bowl of sauerkraut instead. Pickles are delicious. Sauerkraut, in my opinion, is not. Before I had a chance to express my horror, however, my kids started eating it. And they gobbled it all up.

This happened many years ago, and I have thought about it a lot since then. After much scholarly effort, I developed a highly technical theory about why they ate the sauerkraut: They ate it because it was there. And because nothing else was there. If you're hungry and a food is right there, you are bound to eat it. But if two foods are there, it's a battle between them. In a contest between a (not particularly enticing) healthy food and an unhealthy food, the unhealthy food will usually be chosen. It seems to me there is only one contest that a healthy food has a fighting chance at winning: a contest between a healthy food and no food at all.

You don't have to believe my theory just because my kids ate sauerkraut that day. You may even like sauerkraut and find my theory preposterous. But here is some real proof: my University of Minnesota colleagues[31] and I tested it in the lab and in the real world and came up with the same results.[32]

In one test, my colleague Joe Redden told participants that we were interested in their opinions of some cartoons. As you are beginning to realize with our studies, this was a lie. We did not care about their views on the cartoons. But while the participants watched cartoons, we gave them baby carrots and M&Ms to snack on. Some of the people got both snacks at once, and some got baby carrots first, followed by the M&Ms five minutes later. As we expected, people ate more baby carrots when they were alone with them for a while, rather than when they had an opportunity to choose from among vegetables and candy.

We tested the same theory as part of a project to get kids to eat more vegetables in school cafeterias. One obstacle between kids and their vegetables is that they never see healthy food all by itself in most cafeterias—there's always another less healthy and more tempting food right next to it on the tray. We figured that if we could get hungry kids alone with a vegetable, they might eat it. So instead of having kids go right through the cafeteria line when they arrived for lunch, we had them first sit down at their lunch table. Waiting for them in front of each place at their table was a little cup of baby carrots, whether they wanted it or not. We didn't tell them to eat it, or say anything about it at all. On any given day, only about 10 percent of kids at that school chose carrots from the self-serve cafeteria line. But on this day, more than 50 percent of the kids ate the baby carrots we gave them.

We tried this a few more times, partly to see if it would work with other vegetables, partly to see if it would keep working over time, and partly to see if it would work if we gave the students their little cup of vegetables while they were standing in the cafeteria line (since it's not always possible to have kids sit down at a table before they go into the cafeteria). It always worked beautifully. On a regular day in one of the studies, 36 kids ate broccoli. But when we gave them a little cup of broccoli while they waited in line, 235 kids ate broccoli. Overall, kids ate nearly four times as much broccoli when we gave it to them first compared to a regular day. We had even better luck with strips of red and yellow bell peppers. A lot of the kids were unfamiliar with these, but when we gave out cups of pepper strips in the line, five times as many kids ate some, and more than six times as much red pepper was eaten. Even better, after a few days of giving them peppers, they started eating more peppers even when we didn't provide them first. We think they learned to like them.

It shouldn't be hard to make this strategy work for you. There are a few ways you can arrange to get alone with a vegetable. One of the simplest ways to do this is to mimic our approach with the school cafeteria study: start every meal with a vegetable. Meaning, you don't eat anything else until you have eaten your vegetables. The simplest way to do this, of course, is to eat a salad before dinner. Not with your dinner, on the side of your plate—on its own salad plate, before you eat anything else. If possible, eat it before you even prepare the rest of your meal. Eating your salad before cooking the rest of your meal will satisfy some of the hunger you feel before a meal, which will keep you from snacking on the rest of your meal while you prepare it. I don't know about you, but I eat an awful lot of food while I am preparing a meal. If I am grating cheese to add to something I am cooking, even if it is going to be added to the dish in moderation, the amount of cheese I eat off the cutting board often ends up being more than what was going in the dish in the first place. But if I had eaten my salad course before starting to cook the rest of the meal, I would be less hungry while cooking, and would snack on less cheese.

This same strategy applies out of the home. If you're at a party with a spread of finger foods, load up your plate with crudités before you move on to anything else. When you go out to dinner, order an appetizer-sized salad. Ask the server to please bring out the salad first and hold off on serving the main course until you are done with your first course. You may also need to ask the server to hold the bread basket until later, or perhaps not bring it out at all.

There is no downside to eating more vegetables. At minimum they provide all kinds of additional vitamins to your diet. But ideally they will replace other foods that are less nutritious or more caloric, and you won't find yourself face-to-face with a tempting food that you are trying to resist. Take a lesson from Mac Nelson and his slender pig. If it's not there, you can't eat it. What could be easier?

CHAPTER 7

HOW TO TRICK YOUR FRIENDS INTO IGNORING A COOKIE

Last summer, my twelve-year-old son informed me that he would no longer wear shorts that exposed his (perfectly lovely) knees. Not too long before that, my younger son announced that he would no longer eat tomato sauce on his pasta, even though he had eaten pasta with tomato sauce about a thousand times before then. Did my older son suddenly develop fashion sense? Doubtful. Did my younger son's preferences suddenly change? Unlikely. Although both of these boys probably believe they are making fully independent choices, their behavior, like everyone's, is influenced by the people around them. The kids at school were not exposing their knees or eating tomato sauce on their pasta, so my kids weren't either.

In 1956, social psychologist Solomon Asch demonstrated that people conform to those around them when he asked research participants to reply out loud, one at a time, to a very easy multiple-choice question.[1] Although the answer was obviously choice A, the first six students gave the answer B loud and clear. They were secretly in cahoots with Dr. Asch, who had told them ahead of time to say B. But the seventh student was not in on the secret. Asch wanted to know whether this student—and others like him—would give the correct answer or go along with the group. The multiple-choice question was silly and there would not be any consequences to the group or the student if the student gave a different answer from everyone else. Not only that, but the group was made up of strangers that the student did not expect to ever see again. Nevertheless, 75 percent of the students in this situation went along with the group and gave an obviously incorrect answer.[2] The pressure to conform has a powerful influence on our behavior.

People conform to groups in many ways, including in what they eat. Another social psychologist, Muzafer Sherif, said in 1936, "We do not simply eat; we eat certain things, in certain ways, at certain places, and more or less at certain times, all prescribed within limits for a given established group."[3] The group that has the most influence, at least in terms of which foods people eat, is their cultural group or ethnic group.[4] In both Germany and Korea, for example, fermented cabbage is eaten regularly. In Korea it is an ingredient in spicy kimchee, whereas in Germany it is eaten in a different form, as sauerkraut. Nothing prevents Koreans from serving sauerkraut or Germans from serving kimchee, but they rarely do.

Every year I have the students in my Psychology of Eating class go around the room and report what they eat with their family on Thanksgiving. Although many (but not all) of their celebrations include turkey, it was also common to serve additional dishes that are typical of their culture or ethnic group, such as roast duck, adobo, tamales, noodle kugel, pierogis, homemade sausages, or curried vegetables. My family always has chopped liver and kishke at the Thanksgiving table. None of us had ever thought there was anything out of the ordinary about our own family meal, but learning what everyone else was eating demonstrated just how important a role culture plays in food choice. You learn to eat by modeling your behavior on the people around you, without necessarily realizing you are doing it. If your entire family and all of your friends eat kimchee nearly every day, you probably will, too.

In addition to which particular foods you tend to eat, the *amount* of food you eat at a given meal is also influenced by the people around you. This is not always evident, because there are many competing pressures at work when you are eating a meal. Sometimes you may be hungrier than others. Sometimes you may not like the food you are eating. Maybe you don't feel well at one meal, or are in a hurry. But still, the people around you play an important role, influencing your eating in several ways.

One way they influence your eating is by keeping you at the table longer. The longer you are at the table with food in front of you, the more you will eat. I bet you've been in a restaurant and have eaten all you want from your plate, but the waiter is nowhere to be found, so your plate stays in front of you. You invariably continue eating from the plate. By observing people eating in restaurants and recording how much they eat, researchers have shown that the more people you eat with, the longer you stay at the table, and the more you eat.[5] Not only that, but being around people is distracting, so you may pay less attention to how much you are eating, or be less likely to notice feelings of fullness, both of which tend to lead to overeating.[6]

On the other hand, there are also circumstances in which people eat less when they are with other people. This tends to happen in situations where you are highly concerned about the impression you are making, such as when you are on a first date or eating with strangers.[7] Neither situation can be turned into a useful strategy for eating less. Nobody has that many first dates. And how often do you eat with strangers? What really matters is the effect our friends have on our eating, and this is not as straightforward as the effect of strangers. In restaurants, people eat similar amounts of food to the other people in their group, and different amounts than people eating in other groups.[8] But from observing people in restaurants, you can't tell whether one person in a group set a standard that the others then follow, or if the people chose to eat together because they happen to have similar eating habits in the first place.

SMART REGULATION STRATEGY 4: EAT WITH HEALTHY EATERS

To figure out whether friends influence each other's eating, my students and I conjured up the sneakiest study my lab has conducted to date.[9] We wanted to see how people ate around their friends (rather than strangers), but we also wanted to control the situation so that we could tell who was setting the standard and who was responding to it. So we invited groups of three friends to come to our lab for a study on how friends solve problems together. We were not remotely interested in how the friends solved problems; rather, we cared about what they ate while they were solving the problems they thought we cared about.

Before we got the groups of friends settled at a table together to work on the problem, we put them into three separate rooms so that they could have some privacy while they filled out questionnaires. That was our cover story, anyway. We didn't really need to put them in separate rooms to fill out the questionnaires, nor did we even need them to fill out questionnaires. We needed them in separate rooms so we could sneak into two of the rooms and secretly talk to two of the friends. By doing that, we were able to get two of the friends in each group to be in cahoots with us. We told them that they would be offered a variety of snacks when they were solving the problem with their friends, and that when that happened, they should eat only the vegetables. And of course they should not let on that we told them to do that.

Once the two friends understood that they were only going to eat vegetables, we put all three friends back together to work on their problem, and soon we brought in an enormous tray of assorted cheeses, meats, vegetables, and sweets. Each item was bite-size, and each had a colored toothpick in it. We worried it might seem ridiculous that we would provide students with such an incredible spread, so we told them that we had set it up for a special event with a professor and that it had just gotten canceled.

The colored toothpicks weren't just hygienic and pretty. They were also our method of figuring out what each person ate so that we wouldn't have to stay in the room with them, which might cause them to act unnaturally. Whenever anyone ate any of the foods, they would have to leave a used toothpick on their plate, and these were color-coded so that green toothpicks were in vegetables, red in sweets, blue in meats and cheeses. Everyone had a different-colored plate, too, so all we had to do was count each color toothpick from each person's plate.

We were worried that the students would see through our scheme, but that's the one problem we didn't have. In the first group we ran, the students dumped their plates (toothpicks and all) into the trash before we came back into the room. It was easy enough to prevent that from happening again by removing the garbage can. In the absence of the garbage can, one of the students in the next group picked up all the toothpicks and came out of the room to ask us where she could throw them away. We told the next group of students to stay in the room and wait for us to come back. They waited, but while they were waiting, they stacked up the plates and combined all of the toothpicks on the top plate. Since there is apparently no way to stop University of Minnesota students from tidying up a room, we started entering the room a bit before each group's time was up—before they had a chance to disrupt the separate toothpick piles.

With this elaborate setup, we could see what the other friend (the one not in cahoots with us) ate when both of her friends only ate vegetables. As we had expected, when in that situation, the other friend ate more of the vegetables and less of the sweets, meats, and cheeses, compared to participants from other groups where the friends were not restricted to vegetables. If we eat with people who eat a lot of vegetables, our study suggests that we'll eat vegetables, too.

Our eating may also be influenced by our friends when we aren't with them. Psychologists have long known that people's behavior—though not necessarily eating—is influenced by what they think everyone else is doing and by what they think they are supposed to do.[10] These standards or expectations are called "norms," and they have a strong influence on how people behave. For example, if notices are posted in hotel rooms that 75 percent of the guests in the hotel reuse their towels over several days, the guests in those rooms are more likely to reuse their towels than guests in rooms without these notices.[11]

In that example, the norm was specifically stated ("75 percent of guests reuse their towels"). Most of the time, however, norms are implied rather than explicitly stated, but even implied norms are influential. Consider a life-saving example: organ donation. In some countries you are required to sign a form to allow your organs to be donated (called "opting in"), whereas in others you have to sign a form to decline (called "opting out"). An opting-out system implies that agreeing to donate is the norm, and countries with that system have agreement rates of more than 90 percent. An opting-in system implies that *not* being a donor is the standard, and countries with that kind of system have agreement rates around 20 percent.[12]

Given the significant impact of implied norms on such an important decision, we had some reason to expect that implied norms would also affect more mundane behaviors, like eating. We thought that people's eating habits might be influenced by an eating norm their friends had recently implied, even when their friends were no longer present. This would mean they had accepted the norm as their own standard, or "internalized" it.[13] To test that, we conducted a second version of the sneaky toothpick study. This time we provided the most tempting food we could think of: freshly baked chocolate chip cookies, straight out of the oven, with their irresistible smell filling our lab and wafting down the hallway. People in the nearby labs started popping in under flimsy pretenses, suddenly quite interested in our research. As in the other study, we separated our research participants, got two of them in cahoots with us, and told them not to eat the cookies when we brought them in. We assured them that after the session was over we would give them cookies that they could eat. Then we put the three friends back together to solve their problem, and counted how many cookies the third friend (the one not in cahoots with us) ate. Just like in the first study, the friend ate fewer cookies when her friends didn't eat them (compared to groups where the friends did eat them).

The twist to this version of the study was that after the group was done solving the problem that we didn't care about, we separated them again (to complete more questionnaires that we didn't care about) and gave them more cookies to eat alone. That way we could see if the friend who was not in cahoots with us ate lots of cookies now that her friends were gone, or if she continued to resist the cookies according to the norm her friends had just set. Alone in her private room, her friends would never know if she ate any cookies. Even still, the friend continued to resist the cookies.[14]

In sum, once you have learned the norms of your friends, you tend to follow them, even when you are alone.

How to Trick a Child into Eating a Vegetable

Because norms are influential, it is possible to take advantage of them to nudge whole groups of people to do something healthy. In many cases, though, the healthy behavior is not the norm, and this presents a problem. In a study conducted at Utrecht University, researchers explained to their participants the importance of eating fruit, and then told some of them that the majority of their classmates (73 percent) ate the recommended amount, and told others that only a minority of their classmates (27 percent) did. Over the next week, participants tracked how much fruit they ate, and most of them increased their fruit consumption during that time. The only participants who did not increase their fruit intake were those who had been told that a minority of their classmates ate enough fruit.[15] This suggests that if you want people to do something, telling them what other people are doing is only useful if the majority of people are doing it.

When the majority of people are not doing it, it may still be possible to change the norm, but these kinds of broad changes to norms may take years, or even generations. Sushi, for example, is commonplace in the United States now, but in 1985 it was so unusual that in the movie *The Breakfast Club*, one of the characters had to explain to her classmates what the odd-looking food on her plate was. In the meantime, we have to be clever when we try to influence people's behavior based on norms.

In some cases, people are incorrect about what the norm actually is, and correcting their misperception can lead to healthier behavior. For example, college students tend to overestimate campus drinking norms. At one university, students estimated that their classmates consumed more than thirteen drinks per week, when in fact, their classmates were consuming about five drinks per week.[16] Students at that school who were given accurate information about the local drinking norms drank less over the next six months than students who were not given this information.

If you are trying to get kids to eat vegetables, you would prefer they believe an inaccurate norm, because the actual norm is that most kids are not eating vegetables.[17] The tricky thing here is that we cannot misinform kids about the norm. Although we freely lie to adult research participants in our lab (and then explain it all to them afterward), we don't lie to children. It's frowned upon (except with your own children, who, if the occasion calls for it, may be told that Clementine the goldfish has gone to stay at Grandma's house). But allowing children to jump to an inaccurate conclusion is not unreasonable. And that is what we attempted to accomplish in one of our U.S. Department of Agriculture school cafeteria projects.[18]

We did something so simple, it seems to me everyone should do this. We took standard-issue plastic cafeteria trays, which were divided into different-sized sections, and we put a photograph of carrots in one little section and a photograph of green beans in another. That's it. We did not say one word to the kids about it. But we thought the pictures in the trays might give the kids the impression that other kids were using those sections of their trays for those vegetables. That impression was false. Other kids were not using those sections of their trays for vegetables. But we figured it wouldn't matter, because people are influenced by whatever they believe a norm to be, whether their assumption is right or wrong.

To see how much the kids ate when we put pictures in their cafeteria trays, we did the tedious job of pre- and post-weighing the vegetables. We weighed the vegetables on the cafeteria line before the kids showed up for lunch, and then after lunch we weighed the vegetables that were left on the kids' trays. The difference between the pre-weights and the post-weights should be the amount of vegetables that made it into the kids' bellies. Our research assistants soon realized that weighing the leftovers at the fifth-grade table was a more civilized job than having to crawl around on the floor under the kindergarten table, weighing their scraps. (It should be clear at this point why we chose to do this study with carrots and green beans instead of peas and corn.)

All this effort paid off, because we found that the kids who used the trays with the pictures ate three times as much of those vegetables as they ate on a regular day without those pictures.[19] So simple! When this article was published, I got lots of calls from administrators at school districts across the country asking where they could get this kind of tray. But we just used the regular school trays and placed pictures on them. We printed the pictures with a color printer, cut them out, and laid them in the tray compartments. We didn't even glue them down. It didn't take long to do, and any school could do this every once in a while. And every once in a while is how often I think this would work. I don't think this would work if the trays looked like that forever. Then the pictures would fade into the background of stuff you never notice anymore—like the pictures on coins, or the details of your watch face.[20] But every once in a while this could be a useful little boost to get kids eating more vegetables.

SMART REGULATION STRATEGY 5: GET SOMEONE (OR HEY, WHY NOT EVERYONE?) IN YOUR HOUSEHOLD TO CHANGE THEIR EATING HABITS, TOO

We've been talking about how people's eating is influenced by their culture, by the norms among their peers, by their friends, and even by strangers, but we haven't mentioned the people that we eat with most often: our family members and romantic partners. Sometimes our family members have an unspoken influence on our eating. When I am sneaking thin slice after thin slice of Rice Krispies treats from a pan on my counter, I eat a precisely calibrated amount. I eat until right before so much is gone that the people in my household will kill me if I take any more. But unlike cultural factors or norms, which influence us passively, our family members and partners often actively and explicitly try to change our eating habits by, for example, urging us to diet or the opposite—encouraging us to indulge with them. When we instigate changes to our eating habits ourselves, the response of partners and family members can have a large effect on whether we succeed. Being supportive of someone who is trying to change their behavior is not an easy job. Whether that support is effective depends on the partner's motive for helping, the tone of the partner's help, and the type of help that is offered.

There are times when you have a personal goal, and it comes to take on great importance to other people in your life for their own reasons, rather than for your reasons. They want you to succeed not simply because they know it matters to you, but because it matters to them. You might have a friend whose husband wants her to lose weight—not because the husband knows this matters to your friend—but because the husband wants to have a thinner wife. I'm going to go on the record right now saying that I don't like this husband. But aside from that, research shows that people get less effective support—and are less successful in achieving their goals—if their partner's motives are self-focused like this.[21]

If you are trying to change your eating habits, it is helpful if your partner offers encouragement and shows some understanding that these changes are important to you. If your partner (or other family member) nags you, tries to force you to eat (or not eat) certain things, questions or criticizes the food choices you make, or expresses irritation about your choices, you will have a harder time succeeding at your changes.[22] In addition to that, it may become a source of stress and tension in the relationship. It is probably best not to have your partner or family members become your eating police. You may be tempted to ask them to take on this role, but I urge you to resist that temptation. It invariably leads to battles and hurt feelings, and might even compel you to sneak around in your own home or to eat in secret.

The most useful type of help that family members can provide is to change their behavior with you.[23] This is likely to lead to support that has a less nagging, critical, or irritated tone. They won't have to tiptoe through the minefield between being encouraging and acting as the food police. People have a bit more leeway in the kinds of things they can say without offending you if it is clear that they are saying it to themselves as well as to you. I would slug my husband if he were to tell me that I was not exercising enough. But I wouldn't have a problem with him saying that we weren't exercising enough (if he really meant both of us, and wasn't using "we" in that condescending way people sometimes do when they really mean "you"). You don't feel bossed around if your family members are also trying to change their own behavior. Psychologist Maryhope Howland calls this "invisible support" because it does not appear condescending or judgmental, or even like support at all, even though it is incredibly supportive.[24]

It's not only the *tone* of the support that will improve if others in your household are trying to change their behavior along with you. The *type* of support will also be more useful. Imagine you are trying to eat more vegetables by having a salad as your first course at dinner every night. If your family is also making this change, they can help prepare the vegetables, they won't mind waiting for the other parts of the meal, and you won't have to prepare separate foods for them and for you. If you are trying to avoid eating unhealthy foods by keeping them out of sight, it's a lot easier if you don't have to cook those foods for your family. If you are going to use smaller plates to help you eat smaller portions, it is easier if the entire family uses smaller plates instead of you having a different plate from everyone else.

All of the strategies in this book will work better if everyone in your household does them together. And since I am not suggesting that people restrict their eating, but simply aim to live at the low end of their set range, there is no reason why everyone couldn't make these healthy changes. Plus, helping other people—being the giver of social support—improves your mood, and when support is a two-way street, with each person helping the other, your mood improves even more.[25] So instead of causing household strife with just one person making changes, if everyone helps each other do these sensible things, the entire family will be healthier and happier.

CHAPTER 8

DON'T CALL THAT APPLE HEALTHY

've never really understood the classic TV show *The Three Stooges*. Well, I understand the show—the plotline isn't exactly complex. I just don't get why people like it. Seeing someone get whacked over the head with a frying pan makes me cringe, not laugh. I watch the same images that so many of its fans do, but my reaction differs from theirs. This is a very simple example of an idea that forms the backbone of modern social psychology. It's not the particular event we experience that affects how we feel, but rather, it is *how we interpret* the event that matters.[1] That's why two people can experience the same thing, but have a completely different emotional response to it. They interpreted it—thought about it—differently.

Similarly, the way you perceive certain foods affects how you react to them. Food manufacturers know this. If I encounter a tub of vanilla ice cream called Tahitian Vanilla Bean, I am a lot more likely to buy it than if it were simply labeled "vanilla." Is this ice cream really made with vanilla beans from Tahiti? No idea. Is it good to make ice cream with vanilla beans from Tahiti? Who knows? For all I know, all the world's vanilla beans might come from Tahiti. It doesn't matter. Descriptive labels, even when they don't provide any meaningful information, still influence how we think about foods.

To test how people react to different types of food labels, researchers changed the names of several foods in a college cafeteria for a few days. When dishes were given descriptive labels such as Homestyle Chicken Parmesan (instead of Chicken Parmesan), or Grandma's Zucchini Cookies (instead of Zucchini Cookies), students found them more appealing to look at, said they tasted better, and thought they had more calories than those same foods without the fancy descriptions. They also felt somewhat more satisfied and full after eating the fancier versions.[2] You might think the names wouldn't matter since the foods were identical, but they did. They led people to have different kinds of thoughts about the foods, and those thoughts led to differences in their perceptions of the foods, and how they felt after eating them.

Your thoughts about food impact more than your mood—they also affect you on a chemical level. In a convincing demonstration of this, researchers placed intravenous catheters in participants' arms and collected blood samples before, during, and after the participants drank a milkshake.[3] The subjects were given shakes on two separate occasions. On one occasion the milkshake was described to them as decadent, indulgent, and containing 640 calories; on the second occasion it was described as nonfat, guilt-free, and containing 140 calories. Unbeknownst to the participants, they were given the same milkshake each time. But the perceived differences in how they thought about the milkshake triggered a chemical reaction that was evident in the participants' blood. When they thought the milkshake was indulgent and high calorie, levels of the hormone ghrelin—which signals hunger—decreased steeply after they drank it. But when people thought the milkshake was sensible and low calorie, their ghrelin level stayed about the same, signaling that they weren't fully satisfied with the "light" version and remained hungry.[4]

There is of course a biological reason why we have ghrelin—it is there to signal our *actual* state of hunger or satiety, so that we know when to eat and when to stop eating. But this study shows the power our thoughts can have over our biology—the participants' ghrelin levels were influenced not by how hungry they actually were, but by how hungry they thought they were. Thoughts matter. Changing your thoughts can lead to changes in your emotions, your behavior, and as this milkshake study found, even physiological responses in your body. Because thoughts matter, the strategies that follow are all based on the idea of altering them. If we can change the way we think about healthy foods, we may be more likely to choose them. And if we can change the way we think about tempting foods, we may have an easier time resisting them.

CALORIE AND HEALTH LABELS: USEFUL, USELESS, OR WORSE?

If I told you that one slice of pecan pie contains 670 calories—about 50 percent more calories than a slice of pumpkin pie—it might cause you to choose a different kind of pie at your next Thanksgiving dinner.[5] Or it might not have any effect on your pie choice, except that you would feel guilty the next time you ate pecan pie. Or, for some of us, it would just make us want pecan pie even more. The same information changes different people's emotions and behaviors in different ways. For this reason, even though it's generally assumed that providing calorie information on menus will lead people to make healthier choices, it may not.

Since 2010, chain restaurants with at least twenty locations have been required by law to provide calorie information on their menus.[6] It is a sensible-sounding idea, and I firmly believe this information should be available to consumers so they can make informed choices. But dozens of studies have analyzed consumer behavior since this law went into effect, and the weight of the evidence suggests that posting calorie counts has little to no effect on what people order.[7] One particularly rigorous study found no change in the calorie content of orders at McDonald's and Burger King restaurants in Philadelphia when calorie information was added to the menu board, even though customers said they did notice it.[8] At that same time, customers' fast-food orders at the same chains in Baltimore, where calorie information was not provided on the menu, were no different than those in Philadelphia.

Nutrition labels on the back of food packages have not been resoundingly successful in leading to healthier choices, either.[9] Studies have found that consumers may not look at the nutrition information at all, or they look at it without processing it, don't understand it, or are unable to use it to make comparisons among products.[10] Because of these problems, current efforts to make food labels more useful focus on simplifying the information and putting it on the front of packages, where it is more noticeable.[11] Public health organizations, food companies, and researchers have experimented with different kinds of information and formats for displaying it, including, for example, the heart healthy symbol that the American Heart Association[12] has used, or stoplight symbols that are colored green, yellow, or red to indicate the levels of fats or sugars in foods.[13] In Australia and New Zealand they have a system called "Pick the Tick," in which products that are low in fat, added sugar, and sodium are labeled with a tick mark.[14] In the Netherlands, a similar type of label is officially authorized by the government.[15]

The Food and Drug Administration is currently developing a front-of-package label system for the United States based on recommendations from the National Research Council.[16] If the FDA follows these recommendations, the system will provide calorie information plus an overall health score based on levels of fats, sodium, and added sugars. Not surprisingly, there is heated debate between food industry leaders and public health officials over what levels of these substances will be considered unhealthy. The food industry has already spent $1.5 billion lobbying against using a traffic light system, and it strongly opposes putting a red light—indicating a food is too high in fat, sugar, or sodium—on any product, presumably fearing that doing so would negatively impact sales.[17]

Before the FDA settled on a label format, lobbying groups for food producers and food sellers joined together to create their own labeling program, called Facts Up Front,[18] which has been accused of being unduly confusing and not science based.[19] In a head-to-head test, consumers found this format harder to understand and more confusing than traffic light symbols, and were more likely to underestimate the amounts of fats, sugars, and sodium in products that had the Facts Up Front labels on them. Forgive my cynicism, but this may be just what the food industry intended.[20] Regardless of which system the FDA ultimately chooses to adopt, you can expect to hear a lot of screaming from food companies whose products score poorly.

SMART REGULATION STRATEGY 6: DON'T EAT HEALTHY FOOD BECAUSE IT'S HEALTHY

Perhaps the easiest kind of label to understand would consist solely of the word "healthy." But while people do want to know if their food is healthy, the problem with labeling it that way (aside from getting competing interests to agree on which items qualify) is that for many people, the word "healthy" is strongly associated with tasting bad or remaining hungry.[21] In one study, for example, customers at a grocery store were given a cereal bar that was described as healthy or as tasty, and those who were told it was healthy said they felt hungrier after eating it than did customers who were told it was tasty.[22]

Although these results suggest that labeling foods as healthy might prompt people to avoid them, it's also possible that asking people how they feel after eating may not be the ideal way to measure the success of this labeling. The customers might have felt like they were supposed to say they were still hungry after eating the "healthy" bar, or that they shouldn't admit if they actually were hungry after eating the "tasty" bar. We also wondered if the label would matter for foods that people already know are healthy, because much of the time people do already know whether the foods they plan to eat are healthy. So we decided to test the effect of different types of healthy food labels, and to do so without directly asking people how they felt.

We took advantage of a convenient pool of unwitting participants: psychologists from all over the country who were coming to Minneapolis for a social psychology conference. My department was the host for the conference, and as part of our hosting duties, we were providing small hospitality gifts at the conference registration desk. Conferences often give away mugs (which are tough to pack in a carry-on), or tote bags (which nobody needs any more of), or pencils engraved with the name of the conference (okay, fine, these are handy). I surprised none of my colleagues by suggesting that we offer food instead.[23] So when people came up to the registration desk at the conference, we offered them some of our favorite Minnesota-made foods. One was the Nut Goodie candy bar, which is made of nuts and nougat and chocolate and is quite delicious. The second was a source of much local pride, as it was developed at the University of Minnesota itself: the Honeycrisp apple. (At the U of M, people often talk about this apple variety with the same reverence as another local invention: the pacemaker.) The third gift item was a bag of coffee beans from a

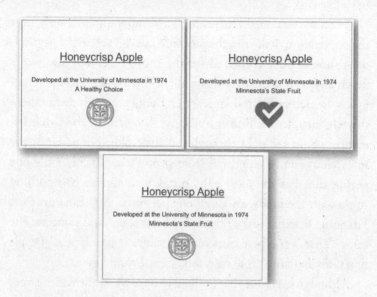

FIGURE 2. Sign with the word "healthy" (top left), the image implying healthy (top right), or neither (bottom).

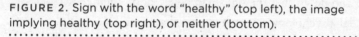

company called Peace Coffee, which is a local roaster that delivers coffee beans by bike, even in the dead of winter.

To test the effects of food labeling, we put signs on each of the baskets of food. For the baskets of Nut Goodies and Peace Coffee, the signs had nothing to do with health, and we left them there throughout the study. But for the basket of Honeycrisp apples, we rotated through three different signs over the course of the conference registration. One of the signs used the word "healthy" (Figure 2, top left). It read: "Honeycrisp Apples. Developed at the University of Minnesota in 1974. A Healthy Choice." On the second sign, in place of the phrase "A Healthy Choice," we inserted the American Heart Association's heart healthy symbol (Figure 2, top right).[24] The third sign contained neither the word "healthy" nor the heart healthy symbol, and it was used for a comparison (Figure 2, bottom).

Then we stationed our research assistants unobtrusively near the registration desk, and they recorded what each social psychologist took as they registered for the conference, and also wrote down any comments they made about the foods. Social psychologists use deception in their research frequently, so it makes them (myself included) a little suspicious. We were worried that everyone would see right through our little ploy, but as far as the research assistants could tell from people's comments, only one person did. For the most part, people's comments had nothing to do with the foods, although one person said, "I can't eat that. I'm going to eat a steak as big as my head later," and someone else said, "This is the best conference because it has apples." People don't say that about tote bags too often, I would guess.

Although everyone that I talked to once the study ended swore up and down that the signs had no effect on their choices, classic social psychology research shows that people are awful at pinpointing the causes of their own behavior,[25] and whether or not they realized it, the signs did influence them. Calling the apple healthy did not lead more people to take it, but using the heart healthy symbol did. About 50 percent more people took an apple when it had the symbol sign than when it had the sign that said "healthy."[26] We don't know for sure why the symbol for healthy worked but the word "healthy" didn't. We don't think the word "healthy" made people think the apple would taste any different from any other apple they've ever eaten. Everyone knows how apples taste, and everyone knows that apples are healthy. They are practically the definition of healthy. It may be that seeing the word "healthy" on the sign makes people feel like they are being told what to do, whereas a more subtle symbol doesn't. People don't like being told what to do, and they sometimes react to that by doing exactly the opposite of what they were told (or think they were told) to do.[27]

We were pleased to find something (the symbol) that did increase people's likelihood of taking an apple and we decided to do another study to confirm that, and to see if we could find anything else that would persuade people to choose a healthy food over an unhealthy one. The conference registration setup had been so convenient that we decided to do the second study at another conference on campus. It was a medical conference predicted to attract more than a thousand scientists. We contacted the conference organizers and offered to provide snacks for all of the conference attendees if they would let us hang around and test different signs and record how many people took each snack. This arrangement was win-win. We got to collect our data and they got to look like very nice hosts.

It was no longer apple season, so we used individual bags of baby carrots as the healthy food, and a local brand of potato chips (Old Dutch) as the unhealthy one. We rotated through a lot of different signs on the carrots over the seventeen hours of conference registration. And we gave away a lot of food. A group of very dedicated research assistants[28] hung out at the registration desks discreetly rotating signs and even more discreetly recording what people took. It's efficient and exciting to collect data on such a large group of people in a two-day period, but it is intense. In particular, the day before the conference, our carrot supplier failed to supply our carrots, and we were left with one afternoon to find and transport seven hundred bags of baby carrots to the conference location. Most stores do not carry hundreds of bags of baby carrots, so my students[29] and I raced from store to store having crazy conversations with produce sellers:

Us: Do you sell bags of baby carrots?
Seller: Yes, how many would you like?
Us: All of 'em.

By going to a dozen stores, we were able to buy enough carrots and disaster was averted. In fact, we had a lot of carrots left over because we mistakenly thought people would take carrots in the same proportions as they had taken apples in the first study. We were way off. About 50 percent of the participants in the first study took an apple, but only about 20 percent of participants in the second study took carrots. Despite that, we still confirmed what we found in the apple study: labeling carrots as healthy didn't encourage people to take them. The healthy sign had no more impact on people's decision to take carrots than a sign that simply said "Carrots: A Snack." But putting that heart healthy symbol on the sign once again led to 50 percent more people taking them. We also tested out signs with other messages, such as "Carrots: An Energizing Snack," or "Carrots: A Snack to Keep You Focused," or "Carrots: A Quick Snack," and people took more carrots when they saw those signs, too. What we learned from people's reaction to these other signs is that labeling a healthy food as pretty much anything other than "healthy" encourages more people to eat it than if you label it as "healthy."

The results of these studies led us to one clear conclusion, which is the basis of Strategy 6. If you want someone to eat something healthy, even something that they already know is healthy, do not explicitly label it as healthy.[30] If you generally regard fruits and vegetables as "health foods" and you tend to avoid them when given a choice between, say, an apple and a bag of chips, try to change your perception of an apple. It is indeed a quick snack, and an energizing snack. Maybe eating one a day really will keep the doctor away—who knows? The important thing is that you come up with reasons that are compelling to you. Maybe you will choose a cucumber because you planted it yourself, or a salad because it has lots of variety, or an apple because it is crunchy and convenient. What we've learned from these studies is that if you reframe the way you look at "healthy" foods you are much more likely to actually eat them.

Health Halos or Healthy Trade-offs?

Not only is labeling or thinking of food as healthy unhelpful, but it can actually backfire. Sometimes the mere presence of a healthy option licenses people to indulge in other ways. In one study, participants tasted bread that was labeled as either healthy or tasty, and then were brought into a different room for an "unrelated study" where pretzels just happened to be available. Participants ate more pretzels after eating the bread that was labeled "healthy" than after eating the "tasty" bread.[31] In another study participants were given either a healthy sandwich from Subway or an unhealthy McDonald's Big Mac, and were then asked to select the rest of their meal from a menu. Participants who were given the healthy sandwich were less likely to order a diet beverage and were more likely to order dessert. In the end, their full meal was less healthy than the meals of people who had been given the unhealthy sandwich.[32]

Researchers refer to this phenomenon as the health halo effect. But it's important to note that there's a fine line between the health halo effect— which leads to overeating when you think you are being healthy—and making sensible trade-offs that allow you to have some balance in your life. If you know you want ice cream for dessert, it makes sense to have a salad as your main course so you can indulge a little after dinner. The trick is getting the balance right so that you don't feel so deprived by your healthy meal that you are tempted to reward yourself in ways that cause you to overindulge. The same is true when people make these kinds of trade-offs with exercise. Exercise doesn't license you to overindulge.

For decades researchers didn't think people could engage in healthy compensation. They conducted studies where they required dieters to consume a milkshake in the lab, thereby breaking their diet, and then asked them to taste-test several flavors of ice cream, which were provided in large quantities. Participants were told that after tasting each flavor, they could eat as much of the remaining ice cream as they wanted. The dieters who had already had a milkshake ate more ice cream than the dieters who hadn't had the shake.[33] It was thought of as a "what the hell" effect. "I already broke my diet for today, so what the hell, I'll have a bunch of ice cream, too."[34]

My students[35] and I thought that study was fascinating, but we wondered if it was realistic. How often are people stuck alone in a room and asked to taste multiple flavors of ice cream from large containers? In their dreams, maybe. But in real life, it would be a very odd situation in which to find oneself, and not many dieters would choose to subject themselves to such circumstances. We also wondered what happened to the participants after they left the lab. Did they continue with their "what the hell" attitude, or did they compensate for eating the ice cream by following their diets more closely?

After years of wondering about this, we conducted our own study to see how dieters would behave in real-life circumstances.[36] We told dieters that we were testing new software for tracking calories, and asked them to use it to report what they ate every day for a week. While we were showing them how to use the software, we were interrupted by a graduate student who was desperately trying to get a few more people to participate in her dissertation study. The graduate student asked the dieter if she would be willing to come back during the week to be in her study. Most of our participants agreed to come back to do this other, "unrelated" study. And of course the other study was not unrelated, nor was it a dissertation study, nor was the desperate graduate student a graduate student at all. She was one of our research assistants, and the other study was our way of getting the dieter to come into the lab and unexpectedly drink a milkshake while she was tracking her calories. That way we could see if she compensated for the milkshake later in the day, or if she fell victim to the "what the hell" effect and continued to overindulge after she left the lab.

Unlike the participants in the classic lab studies, our participants successfully compensated for drinking the milkshake by consuming fewer calories for the rest of the day. When they were free to do whatever they wanted after leaving the lab, they managed to avoid situations that would have required them to be alone in a room with unlimited quantities of ice cream. They tended to have a light dinner and no more indulgences. Our study showed that what many researchers believed to be true for years was missing an important part of the story. When given a choice, people do generally attempt to make trade-offs to balance their indulgences, either by balancing high-calorie foods with lower-calorie foods or with exercise.[37]

SMART REGULATION STRATEGY 7: CHANGE HOW YOU THINK ABOUT TEMPTING FOODS

So far we've discussed how to reframe the way we think about healthy foods so that we are more inclined to eat them. But you may be concerned about the reverse: how can we change the way we think about unhealthy foods so that we are less inclined to eat them? After all, no matter how much we try to avoid temptation, sometimes we find ourselves face-to-face with a doughnut anyway. It's a tough situation, and if we are stuck staring at the doughnut for long enough, the odds of successfully resisting it are slim. But if the situation won't last too long, say if a coworker is walking around offering doughnuts to people and you just need to say one quick no, changing your perception of the doughnut may be enough to successfully resist.

There are many ways to think about a doughnut, and it can mean different things to different people in different contexts. In the present, this doughnut is a burst of deliciousness, but in the future, this doughnut is what may keep you from getting near the low end of your set weight range. Thinking about the long-term consequences of eating the doughnut makes it easier to resist, so think about it that way, instead of thinking about its immediate charms.[38] Not only that, but just thinking about the future *in general* (not even about what eating a particular food will mean to you in the future) can also help people resist temptation. When researchers asked dieters to focus on the future by having them imagine positive events that could possibly happen (such as getting a promotion or attending a party), and then provided them with a meal, the participants ate fewer calories at the meal than dieters who had imagined past events described in a travel blog before eating.[39]

Sometimes your thoughts about a doughnut are specific and detailed rather than abstract or general. It's this particular doughnut, a chocolate-frosted glazed doughnut, a magical combination of fluffy and crispy that will melt in your mouth and leave sugary frosting on your fingers for you to discreetly lick off. Those details are what destroy your resolve. An abstract idea of a doughnut has none of the sensory features that make thoughts of a specific doughnut so tempting. So you should try to think about specific temptations in an abstract way.[40] When your coworker walks by with the doughnuts, instead of thinking about their taste and smell, think about their size, shape, or color. Instead of thinking about that specific glazed doughnut with chocolate icing, think of it as a generic dessert, or even just as one of many breakfast foods. Thinking about the general category makes it easier to resist, at least for a moment, which may be all you need before your coworker walks by. Just as Homestyle Chicken Parmesan is more tempting than regular old Chicken Parmesan,[41] the more you think about the specific features of a tempting food, the more tempting it becomes.

A perfect example of this comes from the classic study of self-control in which children were given a single marshmallow and told that if they could resist it for a little while, then they could have two marshmallows. The researchers trained the kids to think about the marshmallow in several different ways.[42] Kids were more successful at resisting the marshmallow when they were told to think of it abstractly, in terms of its size, shape, or color (for example, "it's a puffy white cloud"), rather than thinking specifically about its taste or smell (for example, it's a sweet, yummy marshmallow).

Not only does focusing on the abstract aspects of a temptation help you resist it, but thinking at an abstract level in general—even if it has nothing to do with any temptations—also helps you resist temptations. It doesn't seem like it should work, but Ohio State psychologist Ken Fujita[43] quite cleverly showed that it does.[44] To get people to think at a more abstract level, he gave a group of participants a list of forty words (such as "dog") and asked them to name a category under which each word could be listed (such as "animals" or "mammals" or "fluffy creatures"). Since a category is more general or abstract than a particular item, naming categories for all forty items on his list put people into an abstract frame of mind.

To get the participants to think at a more specific level, he gave them the same list of items, but asked them to name examples for each one. So for dog, instead of providing the overarching category ("animal"), they would list a specific type of dog (for example, "collie" or "terrier"). After getting his participants to think at these different levels by naming categories or examples for the items on his list, he gave them a choice of an apple or a cookie as a snack. The people that he put into the more abstract mindset were 50 percent more likely to choose an apple than people he put into the specific mindset.[45] Thinking abstractly helped them resist temptation. I'm not saying you should necessarily categorize everything you see the next time a doughnut stares you down, but trying to think more abstractly about doughnuts just might do the trick.

Of course, there will be times when this doesn't work. When changing your thoughts isn't enough to prevent you from eating unhealthy foods, sometimes the best thing to do is stop thinking altogether. In the next chapter, we'll look at some smart regulation strategies that help make healthy eating automatic, so that you do it without even thinking about it.

CHAPTER 9

....

KNOW WHEN TO TURN OFF YOUR BRAIN

If you happen to find yourself walking around Paris, you need to be constantly vigilant or you will find, at some point, that you have stepped in dog poop. It is almost unavoidable, because it is everywhere. The problem is so extreme that every year about 650 people are hospitalized for dog-poop-related injuries,[1] and it is the source of the majority of complaints Parisians make to city hall.[2] In New York, however, this a much less frequent occurrence, even though picking up after one's dog is the law in both cities; the fine for failing to do so is similar in both cities; and both cities have publicized these laws extensively. I have trouble believing that New Yorkers are generally tidier than Parisians, or that they have more delicate senses of smell than Parisians, and I would bet a fairly large sum of money that Parisians don't leave cat poop around their apartments longer than New Yorkers do. So why do Parisians fail so miserably to clean up after their pups?

One possible explanation, if you don't mind me making some broad cultural generalizations, is that the Parisian lifestyle does not make it likely that poop scooping will become a habit, whereas the New York lifestyle does. By "habit" I mean a behavior that is paired with a specific cue in your surroundings enough times that they become linked in your mind, or, in fancy lingo, a mental association forms between the two.[3] Once that association forms, you'll do that behavior whenever you are in those surroundings, without having to think about it or make a conscious decision to do it. It becomes automatic.[4]

In New York, dogs usually stay at home while their owners go to work, so people walk their dogs before and after work, generally in the same place each day. With that lifestyle, scooping can become a habit, because people repeatedly scoop in the same surroundings. In Paris, however, it is not unusual for people to bring their dogs with them nearly everywhere they go, as there are very few places dogs are not allowed.[5] Because of this, they are less likely to take their dogs on walks for the sole purpose of relieving themselves. Cleaning up after a dog cannot easily become a habit with that kind of lifestyle, because the ever-changing poop location makes it difficult to form a link between scooping and a specific location. Without that all-important link, every time your dog visits *la toilette* in Paris, you have to make a snap decision about whether to bother scooping it. And snap decisions are subject to all sorts of interference from your current situation, regardless of your intentions. If you see a cop, or if you notice that the owner of the lawn your dog just used as a bathroom sees you, you will almost certainly scoop it. But if nobody's around, or if you don't see a trash can nearby, you may skip it.

You might also skip it if you think about it too much. Most of us are brilliant at talking ourselves out of doing the things we intend to do[6] (which is why so many gym memberships go unused), so sometimes the best strategy is to prevent ourselves from thinking at all. The strategies in this chapter are all geared toward helping you to behave in certain ways automatically, without conscious consideration or effort. This is smart regulation, because if you do things automatically, you do not have to consciously confront temptation.

SMART REGULATION STRATEGY 8: TURN HEALTHY CHOICES INTO HABITS

One way to make behaviors automatic is to turn them into habits. You probably already have lots of healthy habits. Consider one of the most important things you can do for your health: wear a seat belt. For many of us, every time we get into our car, we automatically reach over and put on our seat belt. We don't have an internal decision-making process. We don't weigh the pros and cons of seat belt wearing four times a day. We just put the thing on. Wearing a seat belt is a healthy habit.

You can create healthy habits around eating in the same way. You can make a habit of ordering a salad in certain restaurants. Once it's a habit, it won't be a decision you grapple with each time you visit one of those restaurants; it will just be something you do automatically. You can make a habit of choosing fruit when you pick up a snack at the grocery store, or of walking through the grocery store without going down the candy aisle. You can make a habit of serving yourself a reasonable portion of food at dinner and then putting the rest away so that you are not tempted to take more later. You can make it a habit to drive a route to work that doesn't pass a bakery, or to walk a route through town that does pass a fruit stand. And you can make it a habit to always buy fruit when you encounter a fruit stand. Once these habits are established, you will consciously face temptation less often.

To create a habit, you need to pair the behavior (say, ordering a salad) with a cue in your environment (such as a certain restaurant). Once you order a salad in that restaurant often enough, the behavior will become automatic. How often is often enough? One study found that once you pair a behavior and a cue repeatedly for two months, it tends to become automatic, and you won't need to think about it.[7] But that's just one study, and as far as I know, no others have come close to quantifying this process. I wouldn't consider two months to be a hard-and-fast rule, and there is great variability between people, and between habits. All we can safely say is that the more times you pair the behavior with the cue, the more you reinforce the connection between the two.

You can also strengthen the link between the behavior and the cue by visualizing the performance of that behavior in that context. I do not mean the hokey kind of visualizing that is popular in self-help books, in which you imagine yourself holding the keys to your brand-new car or successfully achieving some other lofty goal. In fact, that kind of visualizing has been found to make people less likely to achieve their goals, partly by sapping their energy and enthusiasm about trying.[8] There is evidence, however, that if you visualize the *process* of getting to that successful point, including the specific steps involved in accomplishing it, then you are more likely to succeed.[9] That kind of visualizing helps you anticipate and plan for obstacles that may come up, and that is the kind of visualization that may help in habit formation. You might envision serving yourself a reasonable portion of food, wrapping up the rest and putting it in the fridge, and only then sitting down to eat your meal. This won't make it happen, but it may alert you to some obstacles that you will need to overcome, such as needing to find lids for your Tupperware, or having to contend with family members who might want a second helping. It may also help you remember to do the behavior when the situation arises.

Once you have created a habit by pairing a healthy behavior with a cue, you want to make sure you routinely encounter that cue. Now that you always order salad in that restaurant, you should go there often, and now that you always buy fruit when you pass a fruit stand, you should make a point of passing fruit stands regularly. You can also increase how many times you encounter your cue if you choose another, already established habit, as your cue. For example, if you already have the automatic habit of taking a walk at lunchtime, why not create the new habit of walking by the farmers' market? By linking your new habit to your existing habit, you will be more likely to solidify the new behavior.[10]

In addition to forming new healthy habits, you may have some unhealthy habits that you want to get rid of. It's never easy to break a habit (especially a bad one),[11] but one way to fight the "bad" automatic behavior is to consciously avoid the cues that you know are linked to it.[12] For example, if you have a habit of buying candy in the checkout lane every time you go to the grocery store, you may be able to outwit that habit by changing the store you go to, or even by grocery shopping online. If your habit is snacking on the extraordinarily unhealthy[13] popcorn at movie theaters every time you see a movie, you could change this behavior by avoiding the cue—movie theaters. In other settings, people are less likely to eat popcorn, even when it is there. When students were given a box of popcorn in a campus meeting room, they ate only half as much as they ate when they were given a similar box of popcorn in a movie theater.[14] Of course, it would be ridiculous to deny yourself the pleasure of seeing movies in theaters just to reduce your popcorn-eating habit, so instead of changing how often you go to movie theaters, you may be better off trying to link a new behavior to that cue by bringing your own food to the movies.[15] Nearly any food you bring will be better for you than the popcorn there.

The easiest time to make changes to a habit is when you have a big change in your overall environment, such as when you move to a different city. You can link new habits to cues in that city, and you won't have to worry about old habits being cued there.[16] One study found that when college students switched universities, they were able to change their exercise, TV watching, and newspaper reading habits.[17] I have many healthy habits linked to cues in my home, but when I go on vacation, those cues are gone and my healthy habits go out the window.[18] If your habits at home are unhealthy, on the other hand, then vacations may be a time to try to establish healthier ones.

SMART REGULATION STRATEGY 9: CREATE AN AUTOMATIC PLAN FOR ANTICIPATED PROBLEMS

Some behaviors that you would love to turn into habits don't happen very often, so it's tough to create a strong link between the behavior and a cue. For example, most people don't ride in taxis all that often (unless you live in New York City), so there aren't many opportunities to make a habit out of wearing a seat belt in a taxi. Because of that, on the occasions when you do ride in a taxi, you are probably less likely to wear a seat belt than if you were driving your own car. Given the way some taxi drivers drive, if there is one place that you definitely should wear a seat belt, it's in a taxi, so it would be helpful to make that behavior automatic.

Luckily there is an easy way to make behavior automatic even for situations that we don't find ourselves in every day. In fact, it's so easy that you are not going to believe that it works. But it does. All you have to do is create something called an "implementation intention," which is a jargony way of saying a specific plan of action for a situation that you expect to encounter.[19] (It's so jargony that I'll call them i-intentions from here on in.) Suppose you are going to your friend's wedding, and it is going to be a big formal event. There will be a cocktail hour before dinner with roaming waiters offering tempting platters of finger foods. You can easily eat a dozen of these little bites before noticing how much you've eaten. Unless you get invited to a lot of fancy cocktail parties, this situation probably doesn't come up often enough for you to form healthy habits for dealing with it.

I-intentions are the perfect solution. They take the form of an if-then statement that specifies where, when, and how you will handle a particular situation. For example, "If I am at a fancy cocktail party, then I will keep a drink in one hand and a napkin in the other." That will keep your hands occupied and make it difficult for you to grab mini sliders or crab puffs when they are offered. I like this i-intention because it doesn't say you can't have any appetizers, but it makes it just hard enough that you are likely to eat them in moderation. (Remember, humans are lazy. The more obstacles you can put between you and an unhealthy behavior, the better.) No extreme rules and painful denial. Enjoy some appetizers. Just not too many. Here's another i-intention that may be useful in that situation: "If waiters offer me appetizers, then I will eat only one of each kind offered."

To make this strategy work, you need to think of your i-intention before the event, and then simply repeat it to yourself a few times. That's all it should take to make it work automatically during the event. Instead of having to decide what to do on the spot, your decision has already been made. It sounds magical, I know. That's how I felt when I first read about i-intentions, but their effectiveness is well-documented. There are more than a hundred studies that offer evidence that i-intentions work for a variety of behaviors, including things like practicing daily exercise or engaging in safe sex.[20] There is also a lot of evidence that they can help you make healthy food choices.[21] In one study where people were asked to create i-intentions for their meals on a particular day, researchers found that the participants ate more healthy food over the next five days than people who were not asked to set i-intentions for a meal.[22] There is no research on this issue, nor do I intend to conduct any myself, but I bet if Parisian dog owners set i-intentions, the sidewalks of Paris would be a lot cleaner.

The reason i-intentions work is that they help us avoid the common obstacles that get in the way of what we want to do versus what we actually do. For example, one common obstacle is distraction. We tend not to make choices that are in line with our goals when engaged in an absorbing activity (such as watching TV) or when we are distracted in some way. Since i-intentions make a behavior automatic, you should be able to do it even when you are distracted. The father of this research, psychologist Peter Gollwitzer, compares the way i-intentions habitualize behavior to the way you automatically start driving when a traffic light changes from red to green. You don't consciously intend to do it. You just do it.[23] At the cocktail party, even though you are distracted by your friends, you will still be able to stick to your i-intention of keeping your hands occupied, because that behavior is now automatic.

Another common problem that prevents people from acting on their goals is that they don't notice opportunities to do so, or they don't know what an alternative behavior might be in a given situation. When you set an i-intention, you specify the situations you might encounter and what you want to do in those situations. So not only do you have a plan in mind when the time comes, but you are more likely to notice the opportunity when the situation arises.[24] If you hadn't formed the i-intention of keeping your hands occupied at a cocktail party, you might have just written off your health goals while attending it, because you assumed there was no alternative. And even if you did want to make healthier choices at the party, you wouldn't have a plan to make it happen.

Not just any old i-intention will work. Research shows that i-intentions are most effective when they are specific.[25] Instead of "if I go out, then I will eat healthy food," you are much better off with "if I am in a restaurant, then I will order a salad." Researchers have also shown that i-intentions work even better if you first imagine the specific obstacles that stand in the way of achieving your goal, and then devise the i-intention to directly overcome those obstacles. It works just like visualizing your habits, by helping you identify potential stumbling blocks and then devising solutions.

Certain forms of i-intention are ineffective, or can even backfire. For instance, setting a goal to *not* do something rarely works. People ate more unhealthy snacks after creating an i-intention of "If I am bored and I want to have a snack, then I will not eat chocolate!" compared to "If I am bored and want to have a snack, then I will eat an apple."[26] The problem with the negative form of i-intention is that the thing you are *not* supposed to do is put into the forefront of your mind, without a replacement behavior. In this case, being bored puts the thought of chocolate front and center, and does not help you think of any alternatives to chocolate. Because of the ineffectiveness of these "if this, then not that" types of i-intentions, it is not surprising that they do not work as well for reducing unhealthy snacking as they do for increasing healthy snacking.[27]

All you need is one strong i-intention. In her clever dissertation studies,[28] Charlotte Vinkers showed that even having a "plan B" for a situation is not effective. She had some participants make an i-intention for a situation, starting with "if I see chocolate and feel like having a snack, then I will . . ." She had other participants use that same beginning, but come up with two different endings to it. You might think having two solutions to this problem would be better than just having one, but Charlotte found that the participants who came up with two solutions ate nearly 50 percent more calories' worth of chocolate than people who came up with one solution. She reasoned that the strength of the association between the situation and the solutions got split between the two solutions. If i-intentions work by creating a strong link between the situation and the solution, then having two solutions, each weakly linked to the situation, would be less effective than having just one solution that was strongly linked to it. The bottom line is that you are better off creating one strong i-intention for a particular situation than two weak ones.

SMART REGULATION STRATEGY 10: PRE-COMMIT TO A PENALTY FOR INDULGING

There's one other way to prevent your sneaky, rationalizing thoughts from derailing your best-laid plans. In addition to making things automatic so that you don't have to think at all when the time comes, you can also change *when* you think. When the temptation is at a safe distance in the future, you can pre-commit yourself to a costly or unpleasant penalty that will be imposed automatically if you succumb to temptation later. You won't be able to wiggle out of it in the heat of the moment.

This approach can be useful when you are unable to arrange your day so that you entirely avoid temptations. Instead, if you know you are going to be tempted at some point—say, a co-worker's birthday party celebration with cupcakes, or your kid's parent-teacher night with free doughnuts—you can pre-commit to some cost that kicks in automatically if you end up indulging. For example, I briefly used a computer program that was set up to start deleting paragraphs of this very manuscript if I didn't write enough words each day. It was highly effective (until I outsmarted it by repeatedly typing "please don't eat me please don't eat me" until I reached the required word count).

There are many examples of people successfully using this kind of strategy in their daily lives. To force themselves to save, people sometimes choose to put their money in savings accounts that have large fines for early withdrawal, even if those accounts don't have other benefits (like more favorable interest rates).[29] To prevent procrastination, students in one study voluntarily pre-committed to earlier deadlines for their school assignments than their classmates, along with locked-in grade penalties for missing their deadline.[30] In another study, people who were scheduling unpleasant medical tests (and who feared they'd chicken out of showing up) opted to set up a fine ahead of time that they would have to pay if they didn't show up for it.[31]

This strategy was also shown to be successful with families that were trying to eat more vegetables. The families agreed to buy a certain amount of vegetables each month, or else they would have to pay considerably higher prices for all of their groceries the next month. These families purchased more vegetables than families that either didn't agree to be locked into this situation, or that were not given the option to do so.[32] People are willing to lock themselves into penalties for future self-control failures because they know it is good for them, but also because they tend to over-estimate their ability to resist temptations in the future.[33] They don't think the penalty will need to be imposed, so they don't mind pre-committing to it.

Once you get the hang of creating habits, i-intentions, or pre-committing to certain courses of action, you will realize that you can use these techniques to make the other strategies in this book even more effective. For example, you can use each of these tech-niques to help you get alone with a vegetable. You can make it a habit by repeatedly starting dinners in your own kitchen with a vegetable course. You can make an if-then plan about it, such as "If I am eating in a restaurant, then I will ask the waiter to bring my salad before the rest of the meal." Or you can lock yourself into eating a vegetable by packing in the morning only a salad for lunch. It's easier to stick to your goal of healthy eating when the healthy eating is happening later, rather than now. When lunchtime comes, you will be stuck with either eating the salad or being hungry.

You can make most of the smart regulation strategies in this book automatic, and that makes them smarter than they already were, because you won't have to consciously resist a temptation, even if you do happen to get caught face-to-face-with it. It'll happen automatically, even if your mind is elsewhere.

. . . .

CHAPTER 10

HOW TO COMFORT AN ASTRONAUT

For most people, losing weight is a struggle, but there is one known group of perfectly healthy people who are able to lose weight without trying: astronauts. When they spend an extended amount of time in space (at the International Space Station), most astronauts tend to accidentally lose weight. This phenomenon has very little to do with the effects of zero-gravity conditions—being weightless and floating around in a rocket. Astronauts lose weight in space because they don't eat enough,[1] partly because space food isn't the most enticing food on any planet. Many foods are dehydrated before they are sent into space so that they weigh less and stay fresh longer. Those foods have to be rehydrated in space, and while astronauts generally find them palatable, they're nothing to write home about.[2]

There are plenty of space foods that are identical to what we eat down here, but they may still be less enjoyable in space because being weightless causes nasal passages to swell,[3] which makes it more difficult to smell things. This is useful for dealing with space toilets, but it's not ideal when it comes to eating, because food doesn't taste as good when you can't smell it.[4] Even if it did taste as good, you may still get sick of it if you eat it often, which is likely to happen when you are somewhere as isolating as outer space.

Another reason astronauts don't eat enough when they're on a mission is that they're under a lot of stress.[5] They don't like to admit it and they would never complain about it, but they generally have a lot of work to do and not always enough time to do it and meet the high expectations of the people on the ground. Plus there's that nontrivial matter of their lives being in danger, which likely adds to their overall stress levels. As we've discussed, studies have shown that dieters tend to overeat when they are stressed,[6] but astronauts—or at least the nearly two hundred astronauts NASA has studied in recent years—undereat, perhaps because they don't want to take time away from what they are doing.

You might be thinking that this sounds like an added perk of being an astronaut, but it is actually somewhat problematic. While losing five or six pounds over the course of three months spent on the International Space Station is not a big deal, over a longer mission, that rate of weight loss could become unhealthy. And NASA is thinking about a much longer mission: Mars. It takes nine months to get to Mars, and after traveling that far you don't just stay for a long weekend. A Mars mission is expected to last for three years,[7] and NASA is researching all sorts of problems that must be solved before it can even be considered. How do you get enough food and oxygen to Mars? What does three years of weightlessness do to your body? Where do you dump waste? What sorts of people are best suited to handle the isolation and the long journey?

When my colleagues[8] and I heard that NASA was looking for scientists to study stress and eating among astronauts, we jumped at the chance. The idea of helping with the Mars effort was exciting to all of us. Plus, after years of studying people's failed attempts to eat less, I loved the idea of finding ways to help people eat *more*. For several years now, we've been testing ways to reduce astronauts' stress levels and get them to eat more. We thought if we gave astronauts comfort food, maybe we could kill two birds with one stone—they would eat more and get a mental lift.

When you work with NASA, the first step in the research is

creating what NASA calls "ground studies." Ground studies involve only non-astronaut people (who I will, from here forward, refer to as "people"). If the ground studies work, we can then go to the second step, "flight studies." The participants in those studies are the astronauts at the International Space Station.

At first we scoffed at the idea of doing ground studies of comfort food, because everyone already knows that eating comfort food makes you feel better. But when we searched for studies that supported this idea, we found that it was so widely accepted that nobody had ever bothered to test it scientifically.[9] This is exactly the kind of experiment we like to conduct in my lab—one that questions a "fact" that everyone assumes to be true.

To test whether comfort food could fix people's moods, we first had to ruin people's moods. You can't just start with people already in a bad mood, because the bad moods will differ in so many ways that it will be very hard to isolate the effects of comfort food. So we put everyone in the same bad mood by having them watch an eighteen-minute compilation of movie scenes that were carefully chosen to induce strong feelings of sadness, anger, and anxiety. We went through a long, unpleasant process of having our research assistants nominate scenes from movies that they thought caused any of these emotions. If they "worked" on the rest of us, we tested them on students from the Introduction to Psychology class.

Creating these videos was easily the least pleasant task my lab has ever done. The process went on for almost a year—and people were routinely crying in what is typically a cheerful lab. We warned the participants before showing them the clips that they might find them to be disturbing, and we always made sure to cheer them up afterward by showing them a series of funny and happy film clips. Plus we always sent them home with the classic American comfort food: a Hershey bar.[10] Nevertheless, it was a gloomy time.

Once we created two mood-killing sets of film clips, we could finally conduct our study. The plan was to show the clips to participants, and then offer them either a food that they considered to be their "comfort food" or some other food. In order to have participants' comfort foods on hand, we had them complete an online survey a couple of weeks ahead of time. We asked them to list three foods they would eat to make themselves feel better if they were feeling bad, and to be very specific about the brands and flavors, because (unbeknownst to them at this point) we wanted to provide their exact comfort food. We thought it might be disappointing to receive something similar to one's comfort food, but not quite right. I would not be delighted to receive Häagen-Dazs Rocky Road ice cream instead of Ben & Jerry's Marsha Marsha Marshmallow, for example, even though both flavors are chocolate with a marshmallow swirl. One has graham cracker bits and the perfect amount (lots) of toasted marshmallow, and the other has almonds and (not enough) raw marshmallow.

We didn't want our participants to know that the sole point of the survey was for us to figure out what their comfort food was, so we also included a lot of other food questions that were designed to throw them off track. We had them list foods they would eat if they were watching a movie (since that's what they would be doing in the lab), or in a hurry, and in a bunch of other circumstances. Our hope was that by the time they came to the lab for the study, they would have forgotten the details of the survey.

From their list of three comfort foods, we selected one to give them during the study. We couldn't always acquire their first choice. It was not possible for us to provide one participant with her mother's homemade apple pie, for example, or to provide another with a cake that was decorated with a picture of himself. But we[11] managed to get everyone one of their three choices. We also made sure that the food we gave them wouldn't seem absurd to have on hand as a snack after watching a film in the lab. We thought it would seem perfectly reasonable to offer them a piece of cake, or a cookie, or potato chips, for example, but we thought it would seem odd to say, "Please enjoy this bowl of mashed potatoes as a thank-you for taking part in our study."

All of our participants did the study twice (and were shown different unpleasant film clips each time). One time we gave them their comfort food after the film, and the other time we gave them a food that they liked as much as their comfort food, but that they didn't think provided them comfort. If comfort food is really a special thing, then it should do more for your mood than any other food. But it didn't.[12] Comfort food did help people's moods improve some. But the other food improved their moods just as much as the comfort foods did.[13]

This surprised us. We thought comfort food was special. We considered the possibility that only certain kinds of comfort foods would have special powers to improve people's moods. But no kind of food was special. Sweet items, like candy or cookies, did not have special powers. Neither did savory items, like chips. Even chocolate was found to have no special powers.[14]

At this point in the research, we started to feel foolish for comparing comfort food to other foods people liked so much. It seemed like a ridiculously tough test of the power of comfort food, and we couldn't believe we had ever thought it was a good idea to design our study that way. We decided to do the study again, but instead of comparing comfort food to another well-liked food, we compared it to a neutral food: granola bars. We conducted some food opinion surveys and found that granola bars tended to occupy a middle point in people's preferences. They aren't disliked, but they also aren't something people get excited about. Surely comfort food would be more comforting than a granola bar? Nope.[15] As we found with the first study, participants reported that both foods made them feel a little better after watching the film, but comfort food didn't make people feel any better than the granola bar.

We really wanted to be able to tell NASA that our ground studies had worked, and that we were ready to begin flight studies. In our desperation, we conducted one more version of our study, but this time we chose the easiest possible test of whether comfort food comforts. We compared comfort food to *no food at all*. And again, we found that comfort foods provided no special comfort. Participants reported being in the same general mood whether they had eaten after the film or not.

While NASA researchers were also surprised by these results, they still wanted us to test comfort food with the astronauts in space—which, at the time this book was written, we were in the process of doing. A year before the astronauts head out on their missions, they fill out a survey for us that includes questions about foods they like and stressful tasks that they have to do in space. NASA sends them up to the space station with their comfort foods and neutral comparison foods, and then when the astronauts do the stressful tasks they mentioned, sometimes they are given a comfort food, and other times they get a neutral food or no food. The astronauts are asked to rate their moods at certain times and to report how much they eat, so we can see if comfort food brightens their mood more than other foods or no food, and if it leads them to eat more. I hope it does. I hope our contribution to the Mars effort is that the rocket must be stocked with all the chocolate pudding[16] it can carry.

SMART REGULATION STRATEGY 11: DON'T EAT UNHEALTHY FOOD FOR COMFORT

Whether or not pudding has special powers in space remains to be seen—but, down here on the ground, where most of us spend the majority of our time, comfort food does not provide more comfort than other foods, or no food at all. But because it does provide *some* comfort, we tend to believe it is special. We don't think, "I would have felt better even if I didn't eat that," because our minds don't automatically look for scientific control groups. And since we don't expect other foods—say, eggplant—to make us feel better, if we do happen to feel better after eating an eggplant, we don't give it the credit. This is probably why everyone believes in the power of comfort food and why they seek it out when they feel bad. And they do seek it out.[17] When people are in a bad mood, they are more likely to choose unhealthy foods,[18] which most (but not all) comfort foods are. Researchers looked at people's eating patterns the day after their local NFL team played a game. People ate more high-fat and high-calorie foods the day after their team lost (when they were presumably in a bad mood) than on a day after their team won.[19]

We all tell ourselves that we need—even deserve—unhealthy treats when we have endured something unpleasant, or are stressed, sad, or angry. But as our research shows, this is a flawed justification, and it is the basis of Strategy 11: Don't eat unhealthy comfort food when you need comfort. It isn't doing anything special for you. Other, healthier foods you enjoy can provide the same effect. So should foods that are just "meh." Or no food at all. Even if you've believed in the power of comfort food your whole life, it's time to let it go. Comfort food is nothing more than a food you happen to want when you feel bad. So try this next time you feel bad: instead of reaching for the cookies, remind yourself that they will not improve your mood beyond what would happen if you didn't eat anything. Remind yourself that comfort food is a myth. And in fact, by eating something that may make you feel guilty later, you are actually doing the opposite of comforting yourself.

SMART REGULATION STRATEGY 12: SAVOR (NEARLY) EVERYTHING

Even though we know that comfort food doesn't make us feel any better than other foods do, we will probably still eat it sometimes. When you do eat these treats, slow down and take the time to savor them so you don't mindlessly overeat. Pay attention to all of the food's features, noticing its taste, smell, and texture.[20] In fact, why not savor most foods?

I recently had the opportunity to sample lemon meringue pie from a much-buzzed-about patisserie in Paris. I looked forward to it for days beforehand. I ate it slowly and paid attention to every bite. I noticed the soft, pillowy meringue, tart lemony custard, and crumbly crust, and how the ratio of these perfect parts turned the overall pie into something sublime. It was the most glorious dessert I have ever had, and I savored every bite. That pie is more of a special-occasion food than an everyday comfort food, but the point is the same: when you succumb to temptation and eat something you had been trying to avoid, slow down to enjoy it. Sometimes, because you are a human being, you will eat foods that you were trying not to eat, and on balance, I would say it is better to be a human, and occasionally succumb to temptation, than to not be one. But when you eat something unhealthy and delicious that is too indulgent to eat frequently, savor it.

Not only does savoring lead to more enjoyment of the food you eat, but there is some evidence that if you savor your food, you may be satisfied with a smaller portion of it.[21] Remember, part of savoring is eating slowly, so you may feel full before you finish the whole thing. When I was savoring my lemon meringue pie, I did not finish the entire piece (though, to be fair, it was quite a substantial piece). I ate it slowly, noticed that I was filling up, and stopped when I felt satisfied. I didn't want to experience the uncomfortable feeling my son refers to as "being stuffed to the outside."

Another reason savoring may lead you to eat less than you might normally eat is that when you savor, you are focused on your food instead of distracted from it, and distraction leads to overeating.[22] When you are distracted, flavors taste less intense, so people may overeat while distracted because they are compensating for the mild flavor—they need to eat more of the food in order to fully taste it.[23]

In recent years, many experts have espoused the benefits of mindful or intuitive eating, which teaches people to savor food and to pay attention to feelings of fullness and hunger while they eat.[24] There is some evidence that mindful eating may help people lose weight,[25] maintain a stable weight rather than gain weight,[26] or eat a healthier diet.[27] In fact, one of my students conducted a study that found that people who are intuitive eaters eat a more balanced diet (according to USDA guidelines) than people who go on specific diets.[28] Mindful-eating training has also shown promise in helping people with eating disorders reduce their binge eating, and may be a useful tool in helping them recover.[29]

Nothing bad comes from savoring the food we eat, and yet most of us don't do this often enough. Americans, in particular, aren't known for savoring our food[30] (although you wouldn't know it from watching how people eat on TV commercials, with closed eyes and ecstatic expressions on their faces).[31] We eat quickly, often while watching TV, standing over a counter, or driving. French people are known for savoring their food. They eat more slowly than we do,[32] and are more likely to associate food with pleasure than with health.[33] Americans tend to focus on the consequences of eating—what it will do to our bodies—rather than on the pleasant experience of eating.[34]

Interestingly, the Americans who seem to be least likely to savor their food are those who are wealthiest, at least according to one study.[35] And regardless of one's own income, the same study found that simply being reminded of wealth made people savor a piece of chocolate less and reduced their enjoyment of it.[36] Small pleasures—such as delicious meals—may not seem worth savoring when compared to larger, more extravagant ones, and it's possible that people who can have the very best may start to take lesser things for granted.

In addition, there seems to be a trend among the super-wealthy to take healthy, environmentally sound eating habits to the extreme[37] and only consume foods that are some combination of organically grown, locally sourced, small-batch, gluten-free, non-dairy, nitrate-free, air-chilled, grass-fed, and free-range. I am in favor of most of those things, but satisfying a long list of food restrictions doesn't leave you with much to savor. And a world in which we can't savor our food sounds pretty grim to me.

PART FOUR

YOUR WEIGHT IS REALLY NOT THE POINT

CHAPTER 11

WHY TO STOP OBSESSING AND BE OKAY WITH YOUR BODY

Imagine applying for a desk job and being told you are too fat for it, being threatened with deportation because of your weight,[1] or being denied the right to adopt a baby until you lost weight.[2] These are all very real examples of weight stigma or discrimination. The far-reaching consequences of weight stigma include lost educational and employment opportunities, poor medical treatment, and even unfair jury decisions. Taken together, these injustices are far more damaging to obese people than is their weight.

Weight stigma results from negative stereotypes about obesity. Common stereotypes of obese people include being lazy, lacking self-control, and being less conscientious than thin people.[3] There is no truth to these stereotypes,[4] but they do exist, and are endorsed in our weight-obsessed culture.[5] Although most people would never openly admit to being racist or sexist, people do admit to holding anti-fat beliefs.[6] The existence of these beliefs is not only detectable through their outward actions—it can even be observed in their brain activity. For example, in one study, when participants were shown a video of an obese person in pain, they had less neural activity in areas of their brain indicating an emotional response compared to when they watched videos of a non-obese person in pain.[7] Even when we may not be consciously aware of it, prejudice may exist.

DISCRIMINATION

Stereotypes may sound like harmless (though unkind) beliefs, but they become harmful when they are put into action. Discrimination is defined as unfair treatment based on stereotypes or stigma, and weight discrimination is real, pervasive,[8] and has serious consequences, particularly for women.[9] In this day and age, it's hard to imagine being less likely to get into college because of your religion or having to pay more for your employer's health insurance because of your ethnicity—but these forms of discrimination regularly happen to people who are obese.[10] Unlike religion, gender, and ethnicity, which are protected by the law, there is no federal law prohibiting weight discrimination, and only one state (Michigan) and a handful of cities have passed laws that prohibit it.[11] Because of that, victims of weight-based bias have few options for fighting discrimination.

Education is one area in which obese people face discrimination. It is, of course, entirely possible to simultaneously be obese and get good grades in school, yet obese people are less likely to go to college than non-obese people with the same scores on intelligence tests.[12] It's hard to definitively prove that the difference is due solely to weight discrimination, but studies are beginning to show a clear link. For example, one study found that obese people were less likely than non-obese people to be admitted to graduate school if the application process included an in-person interview, even if they had similar GRE scores and grades.[13] If the application process did not include an interview, obese people were just as likely to be admitted as non-obese people.

With very few exceptions, being obese does not detract from a person's ability to do his or her job, but obese people are also less likely to be employed than non-obese people,[14] and the more obese, the lower the likelihood.[15] This pattern is found even when obese people are compared to non-obese people who have the same level of education and job experience. Dozens of studies have been conducted in which participants are shown resumes of job applicants and asked to make hiring decisions. Some of the resumes include a photograph of a fat applicant and others include a photograph of a thin applicant, but the content of the resumes is otherwise identical. These studies have found that the obese applicants are less likely to be offered jobs, even when they have the same qualifications as the non-obese applicants.[16] In one of the studies, an obese applicant and a non-obese applicant were even the same person, just before and after losing weight from bariatric surgery. But participants were still less likely to select the obese applicant for the job, ranking them at or near the bottom of six candidates they evaluated.[17]

A typical reason given for not selecting obese applicants is the expectation that they will have health problems that could interfere with their job performance, but this concern has been shown to be unfounded. Studies that compare obese and non-obese people with similar health still find the obese people less likely to be hired.[18] Some employers don't even pretend that obese people wouldn't be able to do the job, and instead suggest that having obese employees sends the wrong message to their customers. One medical center in Texas refused to hire obese people because they said it set a bad example for their patients, all of whom were presumably slender and in perfect health (aside from being in the hospital).[19]

Obese people are especially likely to be discriminated against when it comes to jobs in sales,[20] and managers have argued that customers' don't like to make purchases from obese people.[21] Whether or not that is true, this is no justification for failing to hire qualified obese people. If a company wouldn't hire African-American salespeople because its customers didn't like to buy from people of color, everyone would agree the company's policies (not to mention its customers) were racist.[22]

Job discrimination doesn't end for obese people once they are hired. They also get paid less than non-obese people for the same-level jobs. This has been shown to be true in multiple studies, and like most outcomes of weight discrimination, women are hit hardest.[23] In one survey, for example, the fattest female participants earned about $29,000 less per year than the thinnest female participants, even when the job level and amount of job experience was equal among the thinner and fatter women.[24] And like the hiring statistics reported above, these comparisons statistically control for health differences that may prevent obese people from performing their jobs. So at equal levels of health, obese people still get paid less than non-obese people.[25]

Discrimination against obese people in education and job opportunities ultimately influences how far they can advance in their career, so it is not surprising that they are underrepresented in positions of power and prestige. Only 5 percent of the CEOs from the 1,000 highest-earning companies in the United States are obese, even though 35 percent of their same-age peers are obese.[26] Obese people are also less likely to be elected to government office. In the 2008 and 2012 elections for the U.S. Senate, there were no obese female candidates, and only 4 percent of the male candidates were obese. On average, the winning candidates weighed less than the losing candidates, and the bigger the size difference between the candidates, the more likely was the heavier candidate to lose.[27]

Finally, although there are no statistics available from actual court cases, a study of hypothetical jury decisions concluded that obese women were more likely than thin women to be found guilty of crimes.[28] Participants acting as jurors saw a mug shot of either an obese or non-obese defendant, and then read a description of their alleged crime. Although the guilt or innocence of the defendant was ambiguous from the description, male "jurors" were more likely to find obese women guilty than they were non-obese women (although they were not more likely to find obese men guilty). Clearly sexism is playing a part here as well. Obese male defendants were not more likely to be found guilty than non-obese males, and female jurors did not discriminate based on weight.

THE EFFECTS OF EVERYDAY WEIGHT STIGMA

In addition to institutionalized discrimination, many obese people are treated with heartbreaking cruelty on a regular basis. In just one week of recording stigmatizing experiences, more than 70 percent of overweight and obese women reported receiving nasty comments about their weight, being stared at, or being subject to negative assumptions.[29] One of the women said that teenagers made mooing sounds outside of a store she was in, and another said that someone told her she must be a bad mother because she couldn't possibly set limits with a child if she couldn't control herself.[30]

Even in the media, obese people are often treated with a level of disrespect that would be considered inappropriate for thin people. For example, a 2013 *Time* magazine cover story about the Republican governor of New Jersey, Chris Christie, offered the double entendre headline, "The Elephant in the Room,"[31] next to an unflattering picture of the obese governor. Christie is well known for poking fun at his own weight, and sadly, laughing along with your tormenters seems to be the socially acceptable response to weight stigma. Nearly 80 percent of obese people in one survey reported using humor in response to stigmatizing experiences,[32] but that doesn't mean they find it funny, and it doesn't mean that this constant assault doesn't take a serious mental health toll.

It is not unusual for obese people to be approached by strangers who inform them they need to lose weight or who offer unsolicited health or fashion advice.[33] Sometimes people are even bold (and thoughtless) enough to remove items from an obese person's cart at the grocery store.[34] Obese people do not need tough love from strangers any more than bald men need strangers sneaking Rogaine into their shopping carts. I probably don't need to tell you this, since it's common sense—but science supports it as well. There is no evidence that bullying fat people leads them to lose weight. Unfortunately, the media[35] and even the academic community seem to think it does, and continue to[36] increase the stigma of obesity in a misguided effort to make America "healthier." For example, a columnist for the *Spectator*, a respected weekly newsmagazine in England, wrote that it is acceptable and helpful to call obese children "hideous lard-buckets," and that "if we don't stigmatize fat people, there'll be lots more of them."[37]

Not only does stigmatizing fat people *not* encourage them to diet, it may actually have the reverse effect. Female college students in one study were asked to read a news article about policies that either discriminated against obese people, or, as a comparison, that discriminated against smokers.[38] Soon after, the students were given a break to watch a film and were provided with candy and crackers as a snack. Of course the students hardly needed a break after the exertion of reading a brief article, but the researchers were interested in how much they ate. They found that overweight participants who read the article about obesity discrimination ate more of the unhealthy snack food than overweight participants who read the article about smoker discrimination. The same group of participants also reported feeling less confident that they could control their eating, or stick to a diet.[39]

Weight stigma does not motivate obese people to exercise, either. Instead, it makes them feel uncomfortable going to a gym and embarrassed to exercise in public.[40] When researchers subtly brought up the idea of weight stigma in one study, overweight women reported feeling less capable of exercising and reduced their intentions to exercise.[41] Among children, being teased about their weight—a common form of weight stigma— makes them less likely to exercise.[42]

Weight stigma can also lead to a physiological stress response. In one study, obese participants who watched a video in which overweight and obese people were stigmatized experienced a spike in cortisol levels.[43] The video was compiled of clips from comedy shows that showed obese people being laughed at, struggling to exercise, and overeating. Since this is how obese people are typically portrayed in the media (if they are portrayed at all),[44] it's fair to conclude that as seemingly harmless an act as watching television can cause this type of stress response for obese people. And don't forget that stress can cause weight gain. So considering diet, exercise, and stress, it's not surprising that weight stigma generally leads obese people to gain weight over time, not lose it.[45]

Sadly, weight stigma is not going away. Even though rates of obesity are rising[46] so that more people know someone who is obese or are obese themselves, the percentage of obese people who experience weight discrimination is also on the rise.[47] With other stigmatized groups, prejudice tends to decrease as more people come into contact with members of that group.[48] But the heavier we become, the less tolerant we seem to be getting of obese people. Even obese people buy into the negative stereotypes about obesity, internalizing the anti-fat attitudes that are

common in our culture.[49] It's hard to rise up against your tormenters if you believe them.

As long as we think of excess weight as the enemy, we are all
complicit in perpetuating weight stigma, and we all suffer for it,
obese or not. Sensationalized reporting of the "deadly" obesity
epidemic makes us view extra pounds as a personal medical crisis,
while misinformation about diets assures us we could have perfect
control over our weight if we would just make an effort. We be-
rate ourselves if we can't keep weight off and judge others just as
harshly if they can't. We feel threatened by people who are heavier
than us, and—thanks to our society's body type ideal, which is
unattainable for most people—jealous of those who are thinner.
It doesn't take a psychologist to see why we are obsessed with
thinness and insecure about our ability to become—or stay—
thin enough.

This is a tough situation to change, but maybe the first step
toward ending weight stigma is to take some of the pressure off
ourselves. If we became a little less obsessed with our own weight,
maybe we wouldn't feel the need to concern ourselves with everyone else's.

BE OKAY WITH YOUR BODY

Allow me to suggest a revolutionary action: Let's try to be okay
with our bodies. I am not saying you have to *love* your body.
I can't help but notice that this goal is frequently pushed on
women, but never men, and if men don't need to love their bodies, it seems to me that women can get by without it, too. For a
long time I bought into all the talk about learning to love your
body, but I've come to think it's a somewhat misguided goal.
Not because it's impossible (though it's difficult for most), but

because it's unnecessary. Perhaps loving your body is something to strive for, but all we really need to do is respect our bodies, appreciate them, and be generally okay with them.[50] Body okayness doesn't mean letting ourselves go, binge eating, or not being physically active. It just means not letting our bodies become our primary life projects.

Historian Joan Jacobs Brumberg researched the diaries of young women around the turn of the century and found that the girls' primary concerns for self-improvement in the 1890s focused on character.[51] They wrote about striving to be kinder and more concerned for others, working harder in school, and rejecting frivolity. One hundred years later, Brumberg found, young women focused their self-improvement on physical appearance, and the way to achieve it almost always involved buying things.[52]

A lot of industries are profiting from our insecurity about our weight and our inaccurate beliefs about how to lose it. It's not just the diet industry. The $27 billion fitness industry (including gym memberships, exercise equipment, and workout programs, among others) is profiting from our ignorance, too.[53] Fitness fads—some more effective than others but none of them free—come and go just as diet fads do. Remember the Bowflex? The Thighmaster? How about Tae Bo? The methods differ but the promised results are the same: we are told that anyone can reshape any part of his or her body. Exercise does many wonderful things, as we'll talk about in the next chapter, but it can't change your build, bone structure, or genetic limits on the amount of muscle mass your body can achieve.[54] If we fail to get the promised result, we end up more anxious and insecure, and eventually move on to buy more and more products.

It doesn't have to be this way. As *New York Times* columnist Frank Bruni wrote in an editorial, "We're so much more than these wretched vessels that we sprint or swagger or lurch or limp around in," and we need to keep that in mind when we resolve to improve ourselves, "foolishly defining those selves in terms of what's measurable from the outside, instead of what glimmers within."[55]

If we take the focus off the outside, maybe we can put a stop to the endless cycle of misguided body improvement efforts and their disheartening and unhealthy aftermath. And if we can take care of ourselves without drama, maybe we can also look dispassionately on other people, without insecurity or judgment. Collectively, as a society, we'd be a whole lot healthier, both mentally and physically.

··································

CHAPTER 12

THE REAL REASONS TO EXERCISE AND STRATEGIES FOR STICKING WITH IT

If you've ever stuck with an exercise program for a while, you probably noticed all sorts of perks. You likely had more energy, were in a better mood, looked great in your clothes, slept more soundly, and perhaps even learned that your resting heart rate or blood pressure had lowered. Exercise offers all of these benefits and many more. You may also have noticed, with some frustration, that you didn't lose a huge amount of weight. You may have thought you were somehow doing it wrong, and that exercise was making everyone rail thin except for you. Despite the weight loss reality shows you see on TV and the infomercials for fitness DVDs that run at all hours of the night, the truth is, exercise doesn't typically lead to dramatic weight loss. Exercise can help you lose weight (especially if you are watching what you eat as well), but the kind of exercise that most of us do doesn't lead to as much weight loss as we would like it to, and certainly not as much as we are told it will.[1] What exercise can do, though, is help you get to the low end of your set range—to your leanest livable weight—and stay there.[2]

One reason exercise doesn't often result in major weight loss is that you have to exercise *a lot* to burn off even one indulgent treat. For example, my standard run takes about thirty minutes. At my (admittedly slow) pace, that run burns about 300 calories—which is fewer than the number of calories in one four-ounce scoop of my favorite ice cream. It's not quite as simple as that, of course. Muscle cells burn more calories than fat cells, so the more muscle you build, the more calories you will burn.[3] But even accounting for that, people may end up consuming more calories than they burn off because they feel hungrier after exercise, or because they tend to allow themselves an extra indulgence on days they exercise.[4] One study found that merely thinking about exercising led people to serve themselves larger portions of food.[5] Even if they don't, it still takes a lot of intense exercise to lead to a lot of weight loss.[6] But that doesn't mean there aren't other good reasons to exercise.

REASON 1: IT REALLY DOES MAKE YOU HEALTHIER

I can't tell you that exercise leads quickly to lots of weight loss, but I can offer better news. The best news, actually. Exercise prevents death. Not forever, of course, but it does increase your life span. Even moderate exercise, including walking (briskly) to work, active gardening, and some kinds of housework, lowers your risk of death.[7] In one study, diabetes patients who walked two or more hours per week had a 39 percent lower death rate than inactive patients.[8] The benefits are evident for exercising just 75 minutes per week, and exercising more often than that, or more vigorously than that, leads to greater benefits.[9]

Even more exciting, perhaps, is the news that exercise works as well as drugs in preventing death among people with heart disease, stroke, or prediabetes, according to a review of 305 randomized clinical trials.[10] The authors of this review compared the effects of fifteen different classes of drugs (such as statins and beta blockers) with the effects of exercise, and they found that exercise and drugs had the same benefits, with just three exceptions. Only one of these exceptions was a drug that worked better than exercise: diuretics for heart failure. The other two exceptions were cases where exercise worked better than drugs (both in preventing death from strokes).[11]

Exercise also lowers your chances of developing major diseases[12] including heart disease,[13] stroke,[14] diabetes,[15] and possibly even colon and breast cancer.[16] Among people who already have risk factors for heart disease, stroke, and diabetes, exercise lowers blood pressure and triglycerides and raises the good kind of cholesterol (high-density lipoprotein cholesterol).[17] And after even a short exercise session, people who suffer from chronic pain are able to tolerate more pain.[18]

Lest you worry that it is too late for you to benefit from exercise, it isn't. One study looked at people who hadn't exercised much before middle age. If they increased their level of exercise and kept at it, they cut their mortality rate in half, ultimately getting the same life span benefits—about two extra years of life—as people their same weight who had been exercising all along.[19] To put the size of that benefit in perspective, increasing exercise in middle age reduced mortality rates just as much as quitting smoking in middle age.

Exercise Helps Even if You Don't Lose Weight

At this point you may be confused. I said that exercise doesn't necessarily lead to much weight loss. If that's the case, then how does it make you healthier? In fact, significant weight loss isn't necessary to reap the health benefits of exercise. This tends to come as a surprise to people, but the evidence is clear. For example, in one weight loss study, researchers were initially disappointed to discover that not all participants lost weight during twelve weeks of intense exercising. A few even gained four or five pounds (and this was not necessarily muscle mass—some had increases in fat mass as well). These differences in weight change didn't occur because some participants exercised vigorously and others slacked off. They all exercised in the researchers' lab, five days per week, for as long as it took them to burn off 500 calories. But when it came to assessing the participants' health, it turned out that weight loss didn't matter—the only thing that mattered was that they exercised. All of the participants showed improvements in heart rate, blood pressure, and fitness levels, regardless of whether they had lost or even gained weight.[20]

The funny thing is, this important news—which I think is headline material—was buried deep within the research article, which was titled "Exercise Alone Is Not Enough."[21] The researchers seemed to be so focused on weight loss that they didn't fully appreciate what was staring them in the face: exercise improves your health whether you lose weight or not.[22] In another study that even more clearly demonstrates this same good news, women were assigned to either exercise or diet for six weeks, and only the women who exercised experienced health improvements, even though they didn't lose weight.[23] The women who dieted did lose weight, but their health did not improve.

REASON 2: IT REALLY DOES MAKE YOU FEEL BETTER

One of the most important reasons to exercise is to help control your stress. I don't know how much stress you have in your life, but I do know you have some. I know this because everybody has stress—especially Americans. We rank 33rd out of 36 developed countries in the amount of time we spend each day on leisure, sleeping, and eating. And unlike our European counterparts, our employers are not legally required to give us at least four weeks of paid vacation each year.[24] In fact, U.S. employers are not required to provide any paid vacation days at all.[25]

Whether the source of your stress comes from your job, your family, your relationship, school, work, money, or your weight, it's important to learn how to manage it, because stress is dangerous for your health.[26] In response to stress, the body's sympathetic nervous system releases the hormone epinephrine (among other chemicals) and raises your heart rate and blood pressure.[27] As we've discussed, this response was helpful when humans needed to flee immediate physical threats, but it's not very handy when you are stressed about a work deadline or an issue in your marriage. Over time, constant activation of the sympathetic nervous system can damage your heart and blood vessels, increasing your risk of hypertension, strokes, and other cardiovascular problems.[28]

And while stress kicks your sympathetic nervous system into high gear, it has the opposite effect on your parasympathetic nervous system, which controls functions like growth, digestion, reproduction, and energy storage.[29] Constantly stopping or slowing those functions can lead to digestive problems (such as irritable bowel syndrome and colitis), and makes it harder for your body to defend against ulcers.[30] Suppression of the parasympathetic nervous system can also lead to fatigue due to depleted energy stores, and since reproductive processes are slowed down, impotence.[31]

Stress also initiates a response that leads to the release of steroid hormones, including cortisol.[32] As we know, cortisol is no friend to weight loss, as it can lead to elevated blood sugar levels and prompts

the body to store fat in the abdomen.[33] Cortisol can also suppress
the activity of your immune system,[34] making you more susceptible
to colds and other immune-related illnesses,[35] slow the healing of
wounds,[36] and maybe even speed up the aging process.[37]

Given how dangerous chronic stress is to the body, reducing
and managing it is important for our health, not to mention our
quality of life. Exercise can help with this, so don't skip your
workout when you are stressed—that's when you need it most!
At minimum, engaging in exercise can distract people from their
worries, and the rhythm and repetition of some forms of exercise,
such as running or swimming, can help relax the mind. In addition, people may also have a decreased physiological response to
stress after they exercise. In one study, for example, after riding
an exercise bicycle for twenty minutes, participants had a smaller
sympathetic nervous system response when they gave a stressful
speech, compared to giving the speech without exercising first.[38]
This appears to work in the long term, too. People who exercise
regularly may be less sensitive to stress overall, not just immediately following a workout.[39]

Most people who exercise have noticed that it makes them feel
good, and this anecdotal evidence is backed by research showing
that even a single session of exercise—as short as ten minutes[40]—
improves overall mood,[41] provided it is not a lot more intense than
what you are used to.[42] It not only works as an immediate pick-
me-up, but it can also change your tendency to feel bad. For example, after being on an exercise program for ten weeks, people report
feeling less anxious in general, not just right after exercising. This
was even true for people who were chronically anxious,[43] as well
as people with panic disorders.[44] Exercise has been shown to be an
effective treatment for mild to moderate depression,[45] to prevent
depression in older adults,[46] and to reduce symptoms of depression
in cancer patients who are completing their treatment.[47]

REASON 3: EXERCISE HELPS YOU THINK, SLEEP, AND AGE GRACEFULLY

Having a regular aerobic exercise program provides long-term cognitive benefits, particularly in memory and executive function,[48] and even a single exercise session can provide a small memory boost.[49] A single exercise session also has immediate effects on creativity.[50] In a series of studies, students were able to come up with more creative solutions to a puzzle while walking—either outdoors or on a treadmill—compared to standing still.

Regular exercise also improves the quality of your sleep, as long as you exercise in the morning rather than the evening.[51] After just four months of regular moderate-intensity exercise, sedentary older adults were able to routinely fall asleep faster and sleep better and longer than their peers who remained sedentary.[52]

The benefits of exercise are particularly evident among older people, even if they had previously been sedentary. Becoming active relatively late in life leads to healthier aging, in terms of preventing chronic disease, depression, disability, and memory impairments.[53] As people age, their muscle mass and muscle strength decline, but strength training exercise can reverse this.[54] Similarly, exercise can also prevent the cognitive decline—in memory and executive function— that tends to occur with age.[55]

MOST OF US DON'T EXERCISE ENOUGH

For a person to get the health benefits of exercise, the U.S. government recommends 150 minutes of moderate-intensity—or 75 minutes of high-intensity—aerobic exercise per week, along with two sessions of muscle strengthening exercises.[56] Moderate intensity exercise is defined as exercise that gets your heart rate up to between 64 and 76 percent of your maximum heart rate (which is based partly on your age and weight).[57] This is more intense than people realize,[58] so it's worth using a heart rate monitor to make sure you are working out hard enough. You can divide the 150 minutes into thirty minutes of exercise, five days a week, or if you prefer, you can divide it into more manageable ten-minute chunks of time. You'll get the same benefits.[59] We've turned the treadmill in my lab into a desk that we can use while walking or jogging. It's too bouncy for writing, but works well for reading, and is a good way to get a couple of ten-minute bursts of exercise into a busy day.

In the 1950s (and earlier), we didn't have to worry about squeezing these bursts of exercise into our day, because without even trying we got more physical activity than we do now.[60] Technology is great, but it has also made our lives too easy. We drive instead of walk, throw our clothes into washers and dryers instead of washing them by hand and hanging them out to dry, and we accomplish a lot of our work without leaving our desks. The proportion of workers in jobs that require very little physical activity has doubled since the 1950s,[61] and jobs that have always been low activity, like my own, have gotten even lower in activity. In graduate school I used to have to walk across campus to the library and schlep heavy volumes off shelves if I wanted to read articles in journals. Now it rarely takes more than a mouse click to access an article.

We haven't made up for this decrease in physical activity from regular daily exertion by increasing the amount of exercise we do in our leisure time.[62] In the 1980s, only 19 percent of women and 11 percent of men in a nationally representative survey reported engaging in *no* leisure time exercise, whereas in 2010 those numbers had risen to 52 percent of women and 43 percent of men.[63] Instead, leisure time is occupied more and more by sedentary activities, particularly, "screen time." Kids used to have to bike to friends' houses to see them, but now they are more likely to connect via their phones or online. Exercise is this miracle treatment, recommended by the American Medical Association, American Heart Association, World Health Organization, and nearly every other medical group you can think of,[64] and yet, people don't take advantage of it.

Well, if you ask people how much they exercise, it seems that they do take advantage of it, but this may be misleading. According to one national survey, about 43 percent of adults met the recommended 150 minutes per week of moderate aerobic activity.[65] In another survey, 60 percent of adults reported meeting the recommendation (with an overall average of 324 minutes of exercise per week).[66] However, when the researchers from this second survey had the same people wear accelerometers for a week to measure their physical activity, it turned out that only about 8 percent met the recommendation (and the overall average was about 45 minutes of activity a week).[67] It's hardly surprising that people overestimate how much they exercise, but I would not have expected such a large gulf between what they said and what the accelerometer measured. No matter which estimate we use (and the truth is almost certainly somewhere in between),[68] there is plenty of room for improvement.

Why Don't We Exercise More?

It's not that people don't want to exercise, or don't intend to exercise. The problem is the gap between what we plan to do, and what we end up doing (and not just with exercise, of course). Across ten studies of people's plans to exercise, about 36 percent of the participants said they intended to exercise but didn't.[69] We join gyms, but then rarely go to them. In fact, 67 percent of people with gym memberships never use them.[70] We buy yoga pants, but end up wearing them around our homes.[71] Why is it so hard to do what we intend to do?

There are so many things that come between our intentions to exercise and our actions that sometimes I think it's kind of amazing that anyone ever exercises at all. For example, some people (I'm thinking especially of new moms) may not have enough time in their daily routine to even schedule a workout. Or they have it on their schedule but something comes up at work, or their kid misses the bus and needs to be picked up, or they forget their exercise clothes, catch a cold, or have an injury from a previous workout. People may not have anywhere safe to exercise, may not be able to afford the equipment, or may not have anywhere to exercise indoors when the weather doesn't allow for outdoor exercise. These are all examples of external barriers—things outside of ourselves that prevent us from exercising.[72]

There are also internal barriers that keep us from exercising.[73] We might be less motivated to bother because we don't feel like we're any good at it, or that it will "work." We may have noticed we aren't losing weight or getting better at the activity itself, or suspect that we aren't getting healthier. Or maybe we can tell that we are getting healthier, but what we really care about is getting thinner. Maybe we don't really think of ourselves as the exercising type, so it's easy to let other things—things that are more central to how we think about ourselves—get in the way of it. Perhaps the people we care about are not fully on board with our fitness plans or don't think exercise should be a priority for us. It may be the case that certain moods keep us from exercising, or make us more likely to exercise.

Some people simply just don't enjoy exercising. It's hard to make yourself do things you don't enjoy doing. Some people love exercise and feel antsy when they aren't able to work out for a few days. It can be hard to like those people, but we shouldn't hold it against them personally, because studies with twins suggest that inherited biological factors may partly explain our motivation to exercise.[74] Although we don't know exactly what those biological factors are in humans, there are some intriguing clues from studies with mice. Researchers took mice that voluntarily did a lot of wheel running and bred them with each other for many generations to create a breed of mouse that is highly motivated to exercise.[75] When they compared those mice to regular, somewhat lazy mice, they found that the fitness buffs had a different neural response to exercise in parts of the brain associated with reward and pleasure. When those mice were prevented from running on their wheel, their neural activity was very similar to that of mice denied morphine (once addicted to it).[76] So for some mice, exercise is extremely reinforcing—perhaps even addictive.

HOW TO STOP WIGGLING OUT OF WORKING OUT

For those of us who aren't that kind of mouse, it can be hard to stick to our exercise plans. Believe me, nobody is better or craftier than I am at finding a reason to skip a workout. Most of the time, though, I am able to keep my lazy side in check by using the same strategies we've discussed for changing our behavior around food. For instance, just like I don't drive to work on a route that passes a bakery when I know I shouldn't stop there, sometimes I change my daily routine so I'm not tempted to skip a workout. If, like me, you tend to be tired later in the day and therefore less likely to make it to your exercise session, schedule it for the morning or lunchtime instead. And just like setting out a bowl filled with fruit makes healthy foods more visible, you can make an effort to keep your exercise gear in your face by packing your gym bag and leaving it by the door. I know someone who actually sleeps in her workout clothes so that she's ready to go first thing in the morning. If you keep your bike easily accessible, you'll be more likely to use it instead of your car for errands. I hate dragging my bike from the shed behind our house, so when I really want to make sure I use it, I lock it up out front instead. Maybe it sounds ridiculous, but tiny obstacles like these matter a lot (remember the smushed toilet paper roll from Chapter 6?).

For many of us, exercise loses the popularity contest for what we want to do in our free time. This is why exercise cannot be entered into that contest. As with eating vegetables first so that they are never in a head-to-head competition with other foods, you can't say, "Tonight I will either go to the gym or go to the movies," or, "This weekend I will either go for a bike ride or go shopping." Your exercise time should be set aside only for exercise. If you don't make it to the gym, then use that time to run errands or do another task or chore you're not particularly looking forward to.

Find a Way to Make Exercise Rewarding

The alternative to punishing yourself for missing a workout is to reward yourself for completing one. For a reward to work, though, it needs to be immediate.[77] If future incentives worked, we'd be fit and healthy already, because we all want the long-term benefits of exercise. Unfortunately, the future benefits do not get us to the gym on a regular basis. We need to be rewarded right away, and often.

For her dissertation study, one of my students[78] gave people a very nice reward for walking 10,000 steps per day: money. The money was indeed a motivating reward for the first week, but once it was no longer being offered, the student participants resumed their normal walking patterns, even though they wanted to stay fit and were continuing to track their steps for the study.[79] The point is: unless you have limitless financial means, tangible rewards are probably not the way to go.

What about if exercise itself were the reward? Just like an apple labeled as "healthy" is less appealing than an apple with a neutral label, thinking of exercise as simply an investment in your health is unlikely to be incentive enough to do it. We need to enjoy exercise. For most of my life, whenever people said this to me, I wanted to bop them on the head and tell them the entire problem was that I did not enjoy exercise. But the best way to stick to an exercise plan is to find a form of exercise that you actually enjoy. This sometimes happens when you least expect it—maybe a friend invites you to try a rock climbing wall with her, or to go to a Spinning class. After a session or two, you find that you're hooked.

Being active without having the specific goal of health or weight loss in mind may actually enable you to enjoy exercising more. When I was under a lot of stress and having trouble adapting to the Minnesota winter, a neighbor suggested I try power yoga. The flowing movements of yoga in a hot room and the soothing words of the instructors helped improve my moods and reduce the chill of the winter. For a while I went mainly for the stress relief, which is a great reinforcer of most kinds of exercise (and a very good reason to not skip your workout when you are stressed). But then something else happened: I began making progress. I started out knowing very little, and practically each session I picked up a new skill—a new pose I could twist myself into, hold longer, or do without agony. It was intoxicating.[80]

You might not love yoga, but the crucial lesson here is that the exercise itself needs to be rewarding, because weight loss comes slowly, if it happens at all.[81] Changes in fitness levels or skills, however, can happen fairly quickly. With yoga, those changes are very noticeable, whether you look for them or not. You couldn't do the crow pose before, but now you can. With other forms of exercise, you might not see changes unless you make a point of measuring a few things. Maybe you will steadily improve how many push-ups you can do, the amount of weight that you can lift, or how far or fast you can run, bike, or swim. Or maybe your resting heart rate will get lower and lower. I highly recommend measuring and tracking your fitness level in as many ways as you can manage.

Another perk of making exercise a reward in itself is that doing so may make you less likely to use unhealthy food as a reward for completing your workout. In two different studies, participants were sent on a walk either for exercise or for the pleasure of listening to music or sightseeing.[82] Even though everyone exerted the same amount of energy on the walk, the people who thought they were walking for exercise ate more unhealthy food afterward than the people who believed they were walking for pleasure. When you change your perception of exercise so that it is something pleasurable, you are less likely to feel the need to reward yourself in other, less healthy ways.

One final way to make exercise rewarding is to make it social—enjoy it with someone else. It's been shown that as with eating habits, other people's fitness habits can rub off on you.[83] If your friends or family members are regular exercisers, you may get swept up in their plans to go hiking, play tennis, or train for a 5K. Research also indicates that the social pressure that you internalize may help keep you on track.[84] For example, if my husband runs a few times when I don't, I feel some pressure to get back out there. Not because he says something. The man's no fool—he wouldn't dare. But his good habits have helped me internalize good habits of my own.

Make Exercise Automatic

The bottom line with exercise, of course, is that we need to make it a habit. We can do that using some of the strategies we used to make healthy eating into a habit. To create a habit we need to repeatedly pair a healthy behavior with a particular setting or cue, and this can be helpful when it comes to your regular daily activities. You may be able to create habits to use stairs instead of elevators in certain buildings, or to walk to certain locations instead of drive. For planned workout sessions, the problem isn't usually pairing the workout with a setting. The problem is getting to one of those settings in the first place. Once you are there, you are pretty much home free.

One way to get yourself to the gym is by creating one of those if-then plans (which we called i-intentions earlier) in anticipation of situations in which you will be tempted to break your plan to exercise. So you might say, for example, "If I am tempted to skip working out because I feel too tired, then I will exercise at a lower intensity that day." This plan is useful because once you start your workout, odds are you will exercise at your normal intensity (and even if you don't, lower-intensity exercise is better than no exercise). The trick is to get yourself to start.

There is solid research showing that creating i-intentions for exercise helps people stick to their exercise plans.[85] In one study, participants were asked to form an i-intention about when and where they planned to exercise that week, to read a pamphlet about the importance of exercise for their health, or to do neither of those things.[86] Reading the pamphlet was no more effective than doing nothing. Only about 35 percent of the participants in each of those groups exercised that week. But 90 percent of the participants who had formed an i-intention exercised.[87] This makes sense, because the problem isn't that people don't believe in the importance of exercise. The problem is getting people to *act* on their intentions to exercise.[88]

In my view, the ideal way to overcome obstacles to exercise is to get locked into a plan. This is harder to do than you might think, since we are, after all, autonomous adults. When people put up the large sum of money for a health club membership, they often think that investment will force them into going. Unfortunately, as is clear from the large percent of people who join fitness clubs and either never go to the gym, or go infrequently, this doesn't work very well, or for very long.[89] The financial investment gradually fades from our mind or we grudgingly accept that it was wasted.

The problem there is that the penalty was paid in the past, so it doesn't motivate us for the future. What may work better is committing to some future penalty now, at a time when your intentions are strong, and then if you violate your plan later, when your resolve is weaker, the penalty automatically kicks in. This is an excellent idea, in theory, and it can work for eating,[90] but it is not easy to find a way to put this into practice when it comes to exercise.

The most effectively I have ever been locked into future workouts was as a member of a novice rowing team. All eight rowers on a crew must show up or nobody can go rowing, so each person is fully accountable to the group. You sign up for workouts ahead of time, when the workout is safely in the vague future and everyone is full of good intentions about exercising. When that alarm clock goes off before the sun rises, rolling over and going back to sleep is not an option, because the seven people who did drag themselves out of bed will kill you. You can't be more locked in than that.

The social nature of that penalty makes it particularly potent. You don't want to ruin things for other people, and you really don't want to make a lot of people furious at you. This is another reason why it can be helpful to have a workout partner. You'll be more likely to show up, and you'll work out at a higher intensity with your pal than if you work out alone.[91] To get that added bonus of feeling locked into the workout plan, you might choose a form of exercise that cannot be done unless both people are there, such as playing tennis. Or maybe your partner can only exercise if you drive her to the gym. That may help lock you into going.

The benefits of exercise simply cannot be denied. Regular exercise can increase your life span, prevent disease, reduce pain, make you less sensitive to stress, improve your mood, aid creativity, help you sleep better, and allow you to age more gracefully. These benefits are more easily attained than dramatic weight loss, and can be yours even if you don't lose a pound. So find a form of exercise you like, and pick a strategy or two that work for you. It really is worth it.

....

FINAL WORDS:
DIET SCHMIET

Someday soon, I'm sure, the diet industry will announce that it has finally found "the diet"—the one eating plan or pill or potion that is easy and pleasant, that makes the pounds melt away, and most important, keeps them off forever. When that day comes, I hope you will calmly observe the hoopla, but keep your wallet closed. A diet like that simply isn't possible, at least not with the current evolutionary state of the human body, the fragility of willpower, and our culture of ubiquitous temptations. Maybe you can lose the pounds relatively easily, but keeping them off would have to become your life's work. And your life is much too valuable to spend that way.

So diets don't work. Big deal. You don't need them to work. You need to not go on them. Should you binge eat, become a glutton, or never eat another vegetable? Of course not. Giving up dieting means eating in a sensible way most of the time, without extensive rules or restrictions. It's a perfectly reasonable thing to do, and nothing bad will happen if you do it. You won't gain a bunch of weight, because your genes will keep you in your general set weight range, and dieting wouldn't get you out of that range anyway. At least not for long.

You can be happy without dieting. And you should. Because dieting isn't merely ineffective. It is also harmful. Not just in the inevitable daily miseries that come with dieting, but in bigger ways, too.

Diets interfere with your thinking ability, lead to obsessive food thoughts, and cause stress, which leads to increases in your levels of the stress hormone cortisol. In high doses, cortisol can cause a multitude of problems, as well as lead to weight regain.[1] By not dieting, you will remove that source of stress from your life.

You can be healthy without dieting. Despite what you hear in the media, obesity will not kill you. Doing healthy things, like exercising, eating nutritious foods, and minimizing stress, will make (or keep) you healthy, even if they don't necessarily turn you into a skinny person.

Here's a perfectly sensible goal: reach your leanest livable weight, that comfortable weight at the low end of your set range. You'll have no trouble reaching it if you exercise regularly and use some of the smart regulation strategies in this book to create reasonable eating habits. The strategies will help you get to that weight and stay at that weight, without expending a lot of effort, without having to endure a life of self-denial, and without having to rely on willpower. Willpower, while quite useful in other parts of your life, is highly fallible, easy to deplete, and simply isn't potent enough to handle the onslaught of tempting foods that you are faced with on a daily basis. The smart regulation strategies don't require you to harness your willpower because again, despite what you may have heard, that has never been shown to be possible. Instead, the strategies just make sure you don't need it.

I urge you to get to your leanest livable weight and then, whatever it is, decide that it's okay. Because your weight is not the point. You were not put on this earth to mold yourself into a perfect physical specimen. As writer Glennon Melton says, "Your body is not your masterpiece—your *life* is."[2] So stop worrying about loving your body and get to work creating your masterpiece.

ACKNOWLEDGMENTS

This book was written during my sabbatical at the University of Cambridge. I am grateful to Theresa Marteau for hosting my visit and for allowing me time to focus on this book. Thank you to Monica Luciana and the Department of Psychology at the University of Minnesota for granting this leave, for being so supportive of my unorthodox work, and for providing financial support for my lab. Thank you also to the departmental staff (especially Liz Gates and Terry Klosterman), and to my social area colleagues (led by Marti Gonzales) for really, truly, letting me off the hook on area duties this year. I'm back on now, I promise.

Gillian Sandstrom, it was wonderful getting to know you and celebrating finishing each chapter with you. I will miss you terribly when I go back home. Thank you to Sara Russo and everyone from the Clare Hall Boat Club for your patience with me; to cox extraordinaire Wilfred Wu for preventing what I was pretty sure was certain death; and to Corinne Benedek for the coffee and conversation, which was often the best part. Thanks also to Gabi Wojczuk at Café Aristo for the motivation to run when I didn't feel like it.

I am grateful to my classmates and professors at Stanford University, where some of the research I describe in this book was conducted, as well as the support I received from the National Science Foundation at the time. Thank you also to the other financial supporters of my work: the National Institutes of Health, NASA, the USDA, the Behavioral Economics and Nutrition

Center at Cornell University, and UCLA. The views in this book are mine, not theirs.

I didn't suffer as much as one is supposed to as an assistant professor thanks to the wonderful environment in the Psychology Department at UCLA. I particularly appreciated the kindness and support of my senior health psych colleagues, especially the women, who were incredible (if intimidating) role models: Chris Dunkel Schetter, Margaret Kemeny, Annette Stanton, and Shelley Taylor (who informed me that as an assistant professor I was done doing housework). And of course, my girls, Yuen Huo, Anna Lau, and Shelly Gable: I still miss you after all this time.

My lab would simply not function without my lab managers: Daniella Pallafacchina, Rachel Shasha, Ashley Moskovich, Jeff Hunger, Anna Larson, Toni Gabrielli, Britt Ahlstrom, Erin Hamilton, Samantha Cinnick, and Lucy Zhou. Thank you for collaborating on this research, and for never making me feel stupid for not knowing how to do expense forms.

To the hundreds of undergraduate research assistants who worked so hard in my lab, running participants through our studies and somehow acting as if I was doing *you* a favor by giving you the opportunity to do so, I am forever indebted.

My graduate students have always been my favorite collaborators, and I have been just plain lucky to work with each of you. Thank you for taking a chance on me, on Minnesota, or both: Kelli Garcia, Erika Westling, David Creswell, Kathleen Hoffman Lambird, Ann-Marie Lew, Janet Tomiyama, Rachel Burns, Heather Scherschel, Mary Panos, and Lisa Auster-Gussman. And welcome to the family, Richie Lenne.

I am deeply grateful to the additional collaborators on the research in this book, including Zata Vickers, Joe Redden, Marla Reicks, Denise De Ridder, Ken Fujita, Elton Mykerezi, Lisa Comer, Katie Osdoba, Barbra Samuels, Jason Chatman, Nikki

Miller, Stephanie Elsbernd, Megan Spanjers, Hallie Espel, Kate Haltom, and Tiffany Ju. I know how much I owe you all, and I tried not to take too much credit here for our collaborative work (though they made me move most names to the endnotes). I sing your praises constantly out in the real world.

To Maryhope Howland Rutherford, dear friend and collaborator, I'm not sure I would have survived my first seven years in Minnesota without your support and friendship. It remains to be seen if I shall survive without you.

To Andrew Ward, my first and longest-running collaborator, people think I am joking when I say that it's fun writing grants, but it *is* fun when I write them with you. I am grateful for your sense of humor and am delighted to battle all reviewers and journal editors with you, plus Godzilla, the Smog Monster, and Lyle Brenner (thanks, Lyle, for comforting me with Bayesian stats), at least until we emerge from obscurity. So there's plenty of time.

Janet Tomiyama, former student, inspiration, and friend: I did not lie or exaggerate at your wedding. I say this without hyperbole: You are a superhero. I shudder to think what my career would have been like had I not opened my office door when you knocked on it. Watching your career has been one of the great joys of mine.

Thank you to the team of experts who kept me from making scientifically dubious claims in this book: Andrew Ward, Hallie Espel, Rob Low, David Creswell, David Sherman, Heather Scherschel, Mary Panos, Jeff Hunger, Janet Tomiyama, and Maryhope Howland Rutherford. Any errors that remain are mine. Special thanks to Britt Ahlstrom, who gave tons of extremely useful feedback on five chapters. Izzy Mann and Corral Johns also gave helpful feedback early in the process.

Two people read every word of this book, chapter by chapter, as I wrote it, and I could not be more grateful. Sabrina Lux, you are a goddess. How you can be so kind, so capable, and so good at literally everything, is beyond me. I am deeply appreciative of the comments you gave me on each chapter, despite being a very busy working mom. Laurie Abkemeier, I feel incredibly lucky that you agreed to represent me. Your willingness to read this as I wrote it, and your sensible feedback and support, have been incredibly helpful to me. You are a rockstar at your job. Thank you also to Julie Will at HarperWave for the insightful, thoughtful, and thorough editing despite being in the midst of wedding planning, and for being on the same wavelength as me about the point and goals of the book.

Like all working moms, I could not manage without outstanding child care. Thank you to the Infant Development Program at UCLA, and our many after-school nannies, including Bambi Laing, Minina Armstrong, Julia Krivi, and Sarah Eckholm. I firmly believe it takes a village, and in Edina, our village includes the clans of Chapdelaine, Huss, Johns, Ruppert, Burbach, and Orzoff, to name just a few. Thank you all, especially for your many kindnesses when my mother was ill.

I am grateful for the three women who have been motherlike to me since I lost my own: Aunt Fran Manushkin, who also gave helpful inside advice about the publishing world; my stepmom, Izzy Mann; and my mom-in-law, Trudie Engel. Also thank you to my extended family. There are too many of you to name, but this includes folks named Mann, Manushkin, Rosen, Levy, Levinson, Adler, Jacobson, Buzil, Krugman, Moos, Novak, Engel, Michels, Banton, and Kanfer, among others. That's right, we're Jews. And while we're on the subject, thank you to Michael Latz and everyone at Shir Tikvah, the most progressive, radically hospitable community in the Twin Cities.

A special mention goes to my cousin Sally Rosen, who makes home still feel like home, and my brother, Barry Mann, who is a constant cheerleader, solid rock of the family, and just a general mensch. I'll sign any document you send me, Bear, without reading a word. Oh, and acknowledging you here? Mom made me say it.

Two beloved family members died between the publication of the hardcover and paperback editions of this book: my grandfather Arnold Rosen, who made it all the way to 101, and like his sisters, Claire and Bernice, was an inspiration right to the end. And my father, Richard Mann, who made me feel special my whole life. The first hardcover off the presses was for him. I'm reserving the first paperback for Oliver Llamas, my dad's longtime and much adored (by all of us) caregiver. Oliver, our gratitude is endless.

My husband, Steve Engel, has been ridiculously supportive throughout my career, and especially while I wrote this book. I'm pretty sure I didn't cook a single meal this entire year, and yet he (almost) never pointed that out or complained about it, despite also dealing with his own highly demanding job. He is the best writer and funniest person I know, and I'm pretty sure this book would have been better if he wrote it (but it would have taken a lot longer, so there's that). Plus, for twenty-three years and counting, he has an unblemished record of not tolerating fat talk.

Thanks to our sons, who are charming, interesting, hilarious, and infuriating. To Ben, my favorite partner in slothfulness, sushi eating, and concertgoing: Your laugh is still the best sound in the world, and your horn is a close second. Except when you make that loud elephant sound in my ear with it, which you are doing *right now*. And to Jonah: I never get tired of seeing the unique and fascinating ways your mind works. You are right and the whole world is wrong: watched pots do boil. I have just one question for you. Okay, a million questions. Starting with the most important one of all: cup or cone?

NOTES

CHAPTER 1: DIETS DON'T WORK

1. Many articles review the mass of short-term diet studies. These are only a sample. Albert Stunkard and Mavis McLaren-Hume, "The Results of Treatment for Obesity: A Review of the Literature and Report of a Series," *Archives of Internal Medicine* 103, no. 1 (1959): 79–85; William Bennett, "Dietary Treatments of Obesity," *Annals of the New York Academy of Sciences* 499 (June 1987): 250–63; Jeanine Cogan and Esther Rothblum, "Outcomes of Weight-Loss Programs," *Genetic, Social, and General Psychology Monographs* 118, no. 4 (1993): 385–415; M. G. Perri and P. R. Fuller, "Success and Failure in the Treatment of Obesity: Where Do We Go from Here?," *Medicine, Exercise, Nutrition and Health* 4 (1995): 255–72; Alain J. Nordmann et al., "Effects of Low-Carbohydrate vs. Low-Fat Diets on Weight Loss and Cardiovascular Risk Factors: A Meta-Analysis of Randomized Controlled Trials," *Archives of Internal Medicine* 166, no. 3 (February 13, 2006): 285–93, doi:10.1001/archinte.166.3.285.

2. For a history of diets, see Wayne C. Miller, "How Effective Are Traditional Dietary and Exercise Interventions for Weight Loss?," *Medicine & Science in Sports & Exercise* 31, no. 8 (August 1, 1999): 1129–34, doi:10.1097/00005768199908000-00008.

3. Michael L. Dansinger et al., "Comparison of the Atkins, Ornish, Weight Watchers, and Zone Diets for Weight Loss and Heart Disease Risk Reduction: A Randomized Trial," *JAMA* 293, no. 1 (January 5, 2005): 43–53, doi:10.1001/jama.293.1.43.

4. According to the fatbet.net website.

5. Paul N. Chugay and Nikolas V. Chugay, "Weight Loss Tongue Patch: An Alternative Nonsurgical Method to Aid in Weight Loss in Obese Patients," *American Journal of Cosmetic Surgery* 31, no. 1 (April 1, 2014): 26–33.

6. The formula for BMI is (weight in kilograms)/(height in meters)^2.

7. K. J. Rothman, "BMI-Related Errors in the Measurement of Obesity," *International Journal of Obesity* 32, no. Suppl. 3 (August 2008): S56–9, doi:10.1038/ijo.2008.87.

8. World Health Organization, "BMI Classification," 2012.

9. The term "normal weight" is a misnomer. Those weights are not the norm, statistically speaking, and the term implies that all other weights are abnormal. I avoid it as much as possible in this book.

10.   For example, see Thomas R. Knapp, "A Methodological Critique of the 'Ideal Weight' Concept," *JAMA* 250, no. 4 (July 22, 1983): 506, doi:10.1001/jama.1983.03340040046030. A long discussion of this issue can be found in Glenn Alan Gaesser, *Big Fat Lies: The Truth about Your Weight and Your Health* (Carlsbad, CA: Gürze, 2002).

11.   Data come from the Metropolitan Life Insurance Company Tables, published in 1983.

12.   Stunkard and McLaren-Hume, "The Results of Treatment for Obesity."

13.   For example: R. R. Wing and R. W. Jeffery, "Outpatient Treatments of Obesity: A Comparison of Methodology and Clinical Results," *International Journal of Obesity* 3, no. 3 (1979): 261–79.

14.   Rena R. Wing and Suzanne Phelan, "Long-Term Weight Loss Maintenance," *American Journal of Clinical Nutrition* 82, no. 1 Suppl. (July 2005): 222S–225S.

15.   Institute of Medicine, "The Nature and Problem of Obesity," in *Weighing the Options: Criteria for Evaluating Weight-Management Programs*, ed. P. R. Thomas (Washington, DC: National Academy Press, 1995), 55–58.

16.   Robert W. Jeffery, Rena R. Wing, and Randall R. Mayer, "Are Smaller Weight Losses or More Achievable Weight Loss Goals Better in the Long Term for Obese Patients?," *Journal of Consulting and Clinical Psychology* 66, no. 4 (1998): 641–45.

17.   G. D. Foster et al., "What Is a Reasonable Weight Loss? Patients' Expectations and Evaluations of Obesity Treatment Outcomes," *Journal of Consulting and Clinical Psychology* 65, no. 1 (February 1997): 79–85.

18.   Weight Watchers has claimed to be more effective than other diets, but studies that compare different types of diets to each other do not support that. For example, see Marion J Franz et al., "Weight-Loss Outcomes: A Systematic Review and Meta-Analysis of Weight-Loss Clinical Trials with a Minimum 1-Year Follow-up." *Journal of the American Dietetic Association* 107, no. 10 (October 2007): 1755–67, doi:10.1016/j.jada.2007.07.017; Dansinger et al., "Comparison of the Atkins, Ornish, Weight Watchers, and Zone Diets for Weight Loss and Heart Disease Risk Reduction: A Randomized Trial.," *JAMA* 293, no. 1 (January 5, 2005): 43–53, doi:10.1001/jama.293.1.43; Bradley C. Johnston et al., "Comparison of Weight Loss among Named Diet Programs in Overweight and Obese Adults," *JAMA* 312, no. 9 (September 03, 2014): 923, doi:10.1001/jama.2014.10397.

19.   R. Cleland et al., "Commercial Weight Loss Products and Programs: What Consumers Stand to Gain and Lose. A Public Conference on the Information Consumers Need to Evaluate Weight Loss Products and Programs," *Critical Reviews in Food Science and Nutrition* 41, no. 1 (January 2001): 45–70, doi:10.1080/20014091091733.

20.   Ibid.

21.   Transcribed from "The Men Who Made Us Thin," series 1. The link was available on YouTube in August 2013: http://www.youtube.com/watch?v=I-_LoAm_etU

22. This 16 percent success rate is higher than anything I've seen in the scientific literature, but it's the number the interviewer used in his question.

23. Lucy Wallis, "Do Slimming Clubs Work?," *BBC News Magazine*, 2013, http://www.bbc.co.uk/news/magazine-23463006.

24. Weight Watchers International, *Business Plan*, 2001.

25. C. Ayyad and T. Andersen, "Long-Term Efficacy of Dietary Treatment of Obesity: A Systematic Review of Studies Published between 1931 and 1999," *Obesity Reviews* 1, no. 2 (2000): 113–19.

26. David W. Swanson and Frank A. Dinello, "Follow-up of Patients Starved for Obesity," *Psychosomatic Medicine* 32, no. 2 (March 1, 1970): 209–14.

27. Two examples are: D. D. Hensrud et al., "A Prospective Study of Weight Maintenance in Obese Subjects Reduced to Normal Body Weight Without Weight-Loss Training," *American Journal of Clinical Nutrition* 60, no. 5 (November 1, 1994): 688–94; F. M. Kramer et al., "Long-Term Follow-up of Behavioral Treatment for Obesity: Patterns of Weight Regain among Men and Women," *International Journal of Obesity* 13, no. 2 (1989): 123–36.

28. That is why financial and other conflicts of interest must be reported at the end of papers. See Frank Davidoff, "Sponsorship, Authorship, and Accountability," *JAMA* 286, no. 10 (September 12, 2001): 1232, doi:10.1001/jama.286.10.1232.

29. We review these studies in two papers: Traci Mann et al., "Medicare's Search for Effective Obesity Treatments: Diets Are Not the Answer," *American Psychologist* 62, no. 3 (April 2007): 220–33, doi:10.1037/0003-066X.62.3.220; Traci Mann, A. Janet Tomiyama, and Britt Ahlstrom, "Long-Term Effects of Dieting: Is Weight Loss Related to Health?," *Social and Personality Psychology Compass* 7, no. 12 (December 2013), 861–77.

30. When we did these calculations, we statistically adjusted the means to account for the number of participants in each study. This is standard practice when some studies are huge and others are tiny. That prevents tiny studies from counting as much as larger ones.

31. As earlier, these means are statistically weighted by the sample sizes.

32. One researcher noted that "greater methodological rigor seems to be associated with poorer results." That is, if your study has none of these problems, it will likely show that most dieters regain the weight they lose. Kramer et al., "Long-Term Follow-up of Behavioral Treatment for Obesity," p. 126.

33. An example is M. Hanefeld et al., "Diabetes Intervention Study: Multi-Intervention Trial in Newly Diagnosed NIDDM," *Diabetes Care* 14, no. 4 (1991): 308–17. Nineteen percent of potential participants were excluded before the study began because they had not been able to control their diabetes with their diet for the previous six weeks.

34. Ranging from 5 percent in one study to 43 percent in another. Author's data.

35. Francine Grodstein, "Three-Year Follow-up of Participants in a Commercial Weight Loss Program: Can You Keep It Off?," *Archives of Internal Medicine* 156, no. 12 (June 24, 1996): 1302, doi:10.1001/archinte.1996.00440110068009; C. Holzapfel et al., "The Challenge of a 2-Year Follow-up after Interven-

tion for Weight Loss in Primary Care," *International Journal of Obesity* (September 13, 2013), doi:10.1038/ijo.2013.180.

36.   M. F. Hovell et al., "Long-Term Weight Loss Maintenance: Assessment of a Behavioral and Supplemented Fasting Regimen," *American Journal of Public Health* 78, no. 6 (June 1, 1988): 663–66.

37.   Robert L. Bowman and Janice L. DeLucia, "Accuracy of Self-Reported Weight: A Meta-Analysis," *Behavior Therapy* 23, no. 4 (1992): 637–55.

38.   G. D. Foster et al., "Psychological Effects of Weight Loss and Regain: A Prospective Evaluation," *Journal of Consulting and Clinical Psychology* 64, no. 4 (1996): 752–57.

39.   T. A. Wadden et al., "Treatment of Obesity by Very Low Calorie Diet, Behavior Therapy, and Their Combination: A Five-Year Perspective," *International Journal of Obesity* 13 Suppl 2 (January 1, 1989): 39–46.

40.   This was corroborated in a survey of dieters. Sixty percent had weighed more than their starting weight at some point since the diet ended, even though only 40 percent did on the day of the survey. Grodstein, "Three-Year Follow-up of Participants in a Commercial Weight Loss Program."

41.   David M. Garner and Susan C. Wooley, "Confronting the Failure of Behavioral and Dietary Treatments for Obesity," *Clinical Psychology Review* 11, no. 6 (1991): 729–80, doi:10.1016/0272-7358(91)90128-h.

42.   K. D. Brownell, "Obesity: Understanding and Treating a Serious, Prevalent, and Refractory Disorder," *Journal of Consulting and Clinical Psychology* 50, no. 6 (December 1982): 820–40.

CHAPTER 2: WHY DIETS DON'T WORK: BIOLOGY, STRESS, AND FORBIDDEN FRUIT

1.   Although many studies do show genes that are involved in obesity. For example: Eleanor Wheeler et al., "Genome-Wide SNP and CNV Analysis Identifies Common and Low-Frequency Variants Associated with Severe Early-Onset Obesity," *Nature Genetics* 45, no. 5 (May 2013): 513–17, doi:10.1038/ng.2607.

2.   Albert J. Stunkard et al., "An Adoption Study of Human Obesity," *New England Journal of Medicine* 314, no. 4 (January 23, 1986): 193–98, doi:10.1056/NEJM198601233140401.

3.   T. Bouchard et al., "Sources of Human Psychological Differences: The Minnesota Study of Twins Reared Apart," *Science* 250, no. 4978 (October 12, 1990): 223–28, doi:10.1126/science.2218526.

4.   There are many twin studies of body weight, but this one is the classic: Albert J. Stunkard et al., "The Bodymass Index of Twins Who Have Been Reared Apart," *New England Journal of Medicine* 322 (1990): 1483–87.

5.   Karri Silventoinen et al., "Heritability of Adult Body Height: A Comparative Study of Twin Cohorts in Eight Countries," *Twin Research: The Official Journal of the International Society for Twin Studies* 6, no. 5 (October 2003): 399–408, doi:10.1375/136905203770326402.

6.   Krista Casazza et al., "Myths, Presumptions, and Facts about Obesity,"
     New England Journal of Medicine 368, no. 5 (January 30, 2013): 446–54,
     doi:10.1056/NEJMsa1208051. In this thorough scientific analysis of diet
     myths and truths, researchers concluded that people's weight (in relation to
     their height) tends to stay in the same general range over their life span,
     and that this is primarily based on their genes, rather than on eating habits
     they learned as a child. One piece of evidence they cited was T. D. Brisbois,
     A. P. Farmer, and L. J. McCargar, "Early Markers of Adult Obesity: A Re-
     view," *Obesity Reviews* 13, no. 4 (April 1, 2012): 347–67, doi:10.1111/j.1467
     789X.2011.00965.x.

7.   The researcher summarizes his own studies in: E. A. Sims, "Experimental
     Obesity, Dietary-Induced Thermogenesis, and Their Clinical Implications,"
     Clinics in Endocrinology and Metabolism 5, no. 2 (July 1976): 377–95. A won-
     derful overall summary of this kind of work is in Gina Kolata, *Rethinking
     Thin: The New Science of Weight Loss—and the Myths and Realities of Dieting*
     (New York: Picador, 2008).

8.   Sims, "Experimental Obesity, Dietary-Induced Thermogenesis, and Their
     Clinical Implications."

9.   Claude Bouchard et al., "The Response to Long-Term Overfeeding in Iden-
     tical Twins," *New England Journal of Medicine* 322, no. 21 (May 24, 1990):
     1477–82, doi:10.1056/NEJM199005243222101. Additional evidence ap-
     pears in A. Tremblay et al., "Overfeeding and Energy Expenditure in Hu-
     mans," *American Journal of Clinical Nutrition* 56, no. 5 (November 1, 1992):
     857–62.

10. This is not because the different pairs of twins engaged in different amounts
     of exercise. Other studies have held exercise constant and still found large
     differences in how much weight different people gained from overeating the
     same amount of calories. James A. Levine, Norman L. Eberhardt, and Mi-
     chael D. Jensen, "Role of Nonexercise Activity Thermogenesis in Resistance
     to Fat Gain in Humans," *Science* 283, no. 5399 (January 8, 1999): 212–14,
     doi:10.1126/science.283.5399.212.

11. A good summary appears in Jeffrey M. Friedman, "A War on Obesity, Not
     the Obese," *Science* 299, no. 5608 (February 7, 2003): 856–58, doi:10.1126/
     science.1079856.

12. Eric Stice, Kyle Burger, and Sonja Yokum, "Caloric Deprivation Increases
     Responsivity of Attention and Reward Brain Regions to Intake, Anticipated
     Intake, and Images of Palatable Foods," *NeuroImage* 67 (2013): 322–30.

13. Kathleen A. Page et al., "Circulating Glucose Levels Modulate Neural Con-
     trol of Desire for High-Calorie Foods in Humans," *Journal of Clinical Inves-
     tigation* 121, no. 10 (October 3, 2011): 4161–69, doi:10.1172/JCI57873.

14. Stice, Burger, and Yokum, "Caloric Deprivation Increases Responsivity of
     Attention and Reward Brain Regions to Intake, Anticipated Intake, and Im-
     ages of Palatable Foods."

15. Jules Hirsch, "Obesity: Matter over Mind," *Cerebrum* 5, no. 1 (2003): 7–18.

16. Erin E. Kershaw and Jeffrey S. Flier, "Adipose Tissue as an Endocrine Or-

gan," *Journal of Clinical Endocrinology and Metabolism* 89, no. 6 (June 2004): 2548–56, doi:10.1210/jc.2004-0395.

17.   Priya Sumithran et al., "Long-Term Persistence of Hormonal Adaptations to Weight Loss," *New England Journal of Medicine* 365, no. 17 (October 27, 2011): 1597–1604, doi:10.1056/NEJMoa1105816.

18.   Ibid.

19.   P. A. Tataranni and E. Ravussin, "Energy Metabolism and Obesity," in *Handbook of Obesity Treatment*, ed. T. A. Wadden and A. J. Stunkard (New York: Guilford Press, 2004), 42–72.

20.   A. G. Dulloo and L. Girardier, "Adaptive Changes in Energy Expenditure during Refeeding Following Low-Calorie Intake: Evidence for a Specific Metabolic Component Favoring Fat Storage," *American Journal of Clinical Nutrition* 52, no. 3 (September 1, 1990): 415–20.

21.   Rudolph L. Leibel and Jules Hirsch, "Diminished Energy Requirements in Reduced-Obese Patients," *Metabolism* 33, no. 2 (February 1984): 164–70, doi:10.1016/0026-0495(84)90130-6. Also see: R. L. Leibel, M. Rosenbaum, and J. Hirsch, "Changes in Energy Expenditure Resulting from Altered Body Weight," *New England Journal of Medicine* 332, no. 10 (March 9, 1995).

22.   Leibel and Hirsch, "Diminished Energy Requirements in Reduced-Obese Patients."

23.   Ancel Keys et al., *The Biology of Human Starvation*, vols. 1 and 2 (Minneapolis: University of Minnesota Press, 1950).

24.   Ibid.

25.   The collaborator was Andrew Ward.

26.   T. Mann and A. Ward, "Forbidden Fruit: Does Thinking about a Prohibited Food Lead to Its Consumption?," *International Journal of Eating Disorders* 29, no. 3 (April 2001): 319–27; Plus a study with kids finds they eat more of a food that was forbidden for just five minutes. Esther Jansen et al., "From the Garden of Eden to the Land of Plenty," *Appetite* 51, no. 3 (2008): 570–75.

27.   Shelley Taylor, *Health Psychology*, 8th ed. (New York: McGraw-Hill, 2011).

28.   Everything I say about stress in this paragraph and the next one comes from Robert Sapolsky's brilliant book, *Why Zebras Don't Get Ulcers*, 3rd ed. (New York: Holt Paperbacks, 2004).

29.   Pamela M. Peeke and George P. Chrousos, "Hypercortisolism and Obesity," *Annals of the New York Academy of Sciences* 771, no. 1 (December 1, 1995): 665–76, doi:10.1111/j.1749-6632.1995.tb44719.x; P. Björntorp, "Do Stress Reactions Cause Abdominal Obesity and Comorbidities?," *Obesity Reviews* 2, no. 2 (May 1, 2001): 73–86, doi:10.1046/j.1467-789x.2001.00027.x.

30.   C. Greeno and R. Wing, "Stress-Induced Eating," *Psychological Bulletin* 115 (1994): 444.

31.   Stephanie M. Greer, Andrea N. Goldstein, and Matthew P. Walker, "The Impact of Sleep Deprivation on Food Desire in the Human Brain," *Nature Communications* 4 (August 6, 2013): 2259, doi:10.1038/ncomms3259.

32.   Rachel R Markwald et al., "Impact of Insufficient Sleep on Total Daily Energy Expenditure, Food Intake, and Weight Gain," *Proceedings of the Na-*

tional Academy of Sciences of the United States of America 110, no. 14 (April 2, 2013): 5695–5700, doi:10.1073/pnas.1216951110.

33. A. Janet Tomiyama et al., "Low Calorie Dieting Increases Cortisol," *Psychosomatic Medicine* 72, no. 4 (May 2010): 357–64, doi:10.1097/PSY.0b013e3181d9523c.

34. Ibid.

35. Diana E. Pankevich et al., "Caloric Restriction Experience Reprograms Stress and Orexigenic Pathways and Promotes Binge Eating," *Journal of Neuroscience{dec63}* 30, no. 48 (December 1, 2010): 16399–407, doi:10.1523/JNEUROSCI.1955-10.2010.

36. Jeffrey Friedman, cited on page 125 of Kolata, *Rethinking Thin*.

CHAPTER 3: THE MYTH OF WILLPOWER

1. Sorbet is usually lower in sugars and carbohydrates than ice cream but just a little bit lower, so if you are trying to reduce those, sorbet might not be the most helpful choice for you.

2. K. D. Brownell and K. B. Horgen, *Food Fight: The Inside Story of the Food Industry, America's Obesity Crisis, and What We Can Do About It* (Chicago: Contemporary Books, 2004). Brownell refers to this environment as a "toxic food environment."

3. For the argument that fats and sugars cause cravings for more fats and sugars, and that the food industry has taken advantage of this, see D. A. Kessler, *The End of Overeating: Taking Control of the Insatiable American Appetite* (Emmaus, PA: Rodale, 2009).

4. John P. Foreyt and G. Ken Goodrick, *Living Without Dieting* (New York: Grand Central, 1994).

5. The most commonly used questionnaire for measuring self-control can be found in J. Tangney, R. Baumeister, and A. Boone, "High Self-Control Predicts Good Adjustment, Less Pathology, Better Grades, and Interpersonal Success," *Journal of Personality* 72, no. 2 (2004): 271–324.

6. M. Friese and W. Hofmann, "Control Me or I Will Control You: Impulses, Trait Self-Control, and the Guidance of Behavior," *Journal of Research in Personality* (2009).

7. They did a much better job than we did, which is why our study was never published, but theirs was: Denise T. D. de Ridder et al., "Taking Stock of Self-Control: A Meta-Analysis of How Trait Self-Control Relates to a Wide Range of Behaviors," *Personality and Social Psychology Review* 16, no. 1 (February 1, 2012): 76–99, doi:10.1177/1088868311418749.

8. Brandon J. Schmeichel and Anne Zell, "Trait Self-Control Predicts Performance on Behavioral Tests of Self-Control," *Journal of Personality* 75, no. 4 (August 2007): 743–55, doi:10.1111/j.1467-6494.2007.00455.x.

9. Walter Mischel and Ebbe Ebbesen, "Attention in Delay of Gratification," *Journal of Personality and Social Psychology* 16, no. 2 (1970): 329–37.

10. The stress and frustration findings are in W. Mischel, Y. Shoda, and P. K.

Peake, "The Nature of Adolescent Competencies Predicted by Preschool Delay of Gratification," *Journal of Personality and Social Psychology* 54, no. 4 (April 1988): 687–96. A review of many findings from that line of research is in W. Mischel, Y. Shoda, and M. Rodriguez, "Delay of Gratification in Children," *Choice over Time* (New York: Russell Sage Foundation, 1992), 147–64.

11.   Body mass index is a measure of weight that takes height into account.

12.   Tanya R. Schlam et al., "Preschoolers' Delay of Gratification Predicts Their Body Mass 30 Years Later," *Journal of Pediatrics* 162, no. 1 (January 2013): 90–93, doi:10.1016/j.jpeds.2012.06.049. The fact that there is any relationship whatsoever to behavior that occurs thirty years later is remarkable, but the delay of gratification test explains only about 4 percent of the differences between people's weights, leaving the other 96 percent to be accounted for by other things.

13.   Other studies have used that same kind of test and found similarly small relationships, and once researchers control for common confounding factors, they tend to disappear. For example, see the following studies for, in order, a similar small relationship, an even smaller one, and no relationship at all. Lori A. Francis and Elizabeth J. Susman, "Self-Regulation and Rapid Weight Gain in Children from Age 3 to 12 Years," *Archives of Pediatrics & Adolescent Medicine* 163, no. 4 (April 6, 2009): 297–302, doi:10.1001/archpediatrics.2008.579; Angela L. Duckworth, Eli Tsukayama, and Andrew B. Geier, "Self-Controlled Children Stay Leaner in the Transition to Adolescence," *Appetite* 54, no. 2 (2010): 304–8; Desiree M Seeyave et al., "Ability to Delay Gratification at Age 4 Years and Risk of Overweight at Age 11 Years," *Archives of Pediatrics & Adolescent Medicine* 163, no. 4 (April 6, 2009): 303–8, doi:10.1001/archpediatrics.2009.12.

14.   Joseph P. Redden and Kelly Haws, "Healthy Satiation: The Role of Decreasing Desire in Effective Self-Control" (October 25, 2012).

15.   Nicholas Carr, *The Shallows: What the Internet Is Doing to Our Brains* (New York: Norton, 2011).

16.   Larry D. Rosen, L. Mark Carrier, and Nancy A. Cheever, "Facebook and Texting Made Me Do It: Media-Induced Task-Switching While Studying," *Computers in Human Behavior* 29, no. 3 (May 2013): 948–58, doi:10.1016/j.chb.2012.12.001.

17.   Andrew Ward and Traci Mann, "Don't Mind If I Do: Disinhibited Eating under Cognitive Load," *Journal of Personality and Social Psychology* 78, no. 4 (April 1, 2000): 753–63, doi:10.1037//0022-3514.78.4.753.

18.   Philip G. Zimbardo, "On the Ethics of Intervention in Human Psychological Research: With Special Reference to the Stanford Prison Experiment," *Cognition* 2, no. 2 (January 1973): 243–56.

19.   J. Polivy and C. P. Herman, "Effects of Alcohol on Eating Behavior: Influence of Mood and Perceived Intoxication," *Journal of Abnormal Psychology* 85, no. 6 (December 1976): 601–6.

20.   This idea comes from our professor Claude Steele's work on alcohol my-

opia, described in C. M. Steele and R. A. Josephs, "Alcohol Myopia: Its Prized and Dangerous Effects," *American Psychologist* 45, no. 8 (August 1990): 921–33.

21. Plus we have to justify to the university's Institutional Review Board why we are using deception, and show that we are using as little of it as possible.

22. This is the classic example: C. Peter Herman and Deborah Mack, "Restrained and Unrestrained Eating," *Journal of Personality* 43, no. 4 (December 1975): 647–60, doi:10.1111/j.1467-6494.1975.tb00727.x.

23. Seven studies of this are shown in Greeno and Wing, "Stress-Induced Eating." And there have been many more since then.

24. C. Peter Herman and Janet Polivy, "Anxiety, Restraint, and Eating Behavior," *Journal of Abnormal Psychology* 84, no. 6 (1975): 666–72, doi:10.1037/0021 843X.84.6.666.

25. Two examples: Elissa Epel et al., "Stress May Add Bite to Appetite in Women: A Laboratory Study of Stress-Induced Cortisol and Eating Behavior," *Psychoneuroendocrinology* 26, no. 1 (January 2001): 37–49, doi:10.1016/ S0306-4530(00)00035-4; Summar Habhab, Jane P. Sheldon, and Roger C. Loeb, "The Relationship between Stress, Dietary Restraint, and Food Preferences in Women," *Appetite* 52, no. 2 (April 2009): 437–44, doi:10.1016/j .appet.2008.12.006.

26. J. Cools, D. E. Schotte, and R. J. McNally, "Emotional Arousal and Overeating in Restrained Eaters," *Journal of Abnormal Psychology* 101, no. 2 (May 1992): 348–51.

27. A. Janet Tomiyama, Traci Mann, and Lisa Comer, "Triggers of Eating in Everyday Life," *Appetite* 52, no. 1 (2009): 72–82.

28. Eighty-three separate studies are cited in Martin S. Hagger et al., "Ego Depletion and the Strength Model of Self-Control: A Meta-Analysis," *Psychological Bulletin* 136, no. 4 (July 2010): 495–525, doi:10.1037/a0019486.

29. This is the original study of this phenomenon: Roy F. Baumeister et al., "Ego Depletion: Is the Active Self a Limited Resource?," *Journal of Personality and Social Psychology* 74, no. 5 (1998): 1252–65, doi:10.1037/002 2-3514.74.5.1252.

30. All of these are cited in Hagger et al., "Ego Depletion and the Strength Model of Self-Control: A Meta-Analysis."

31. The many downsides of having too much choice are covered beautifully in Barry Schwartz, *The Paradox of Choice*, (New York: Ecco, 2003).

32. S. S. Iyengar and M. R. Lepper, "When Choice Is Demotivating: Can One Desire Too Much of a Good Thing?," *Journal of Personality and Social Psychology* 79, no. 6 (December 2000): 995–1006.

33. Kathleen D. Vohs et al., "Making Choices Impairs Subsequent Self-Control: A Limited-Resource Account of Decision Making, Self-Regulation, and Active Initiative," *Journal of Personality and Social Psychology* 94, no. 5 (May 2008): 883–98, doi:10.1037/0022-3514.94.5.883.

34. Michael Lewis, "Obama's Way," *Vanity Fair*, 2012.

35. See, for example, Roy F. Baumeister and John Tierney, *Willpower: Rediscov-

ering the Greatest Human Strength (New York: Penguin Books, 2012).

36. These articles seem a bit peripheral to the issue. Instead of teaching self-regulation, they have participants do things like control their posture or engage in an exercise program, and then show that they can control *something else* better. In addition, they are riddled with methodological problems that would keep a research methods class busy for hours. M. Muraven, R. F. Baumeister, and D. M. Tice, "Longitudinal Improvement of Self-Regulation Through Practice: Building Self-Control Strength Through Repeated Exercise," *Journal of Social Psychology* 139, no. 4 (August 1999): 446–57, doi:10.1080/00224549909598404; Megan Oaten and Ken Cheng, "Improved Self-Control: The Benefits of a Regular Program of Academic Study," *Basic and Applied Social Psychology* 28, no. 1 (April 2006): 1–16, doi:10.1207/s15324834basp2801_1; Megan Oaten and Ken Cheng, "Longitudinal Gains in Self-Regulation from Regular Physical Exercise," *British Journal of Health Psychology* 11, Pt. 4 (November 2006): 717–33, doi:10.1348/135910706X96481.

37. Dutch self-control researcher Denise De Ridder introduced me to this saying. It is also common in Gaelic.

38. See, for example, Wilhelm Hofmann et al., "Everyday Temptations: An Experience Sampling Study of Desire, Conflict, and Self-Control," *Journal of Personality and Social Psychology* 102, no. 6 (June 2012): 1318–35, doi:10.1037/a0026545.

CHAPTER 4: DIETS ARE BAD FOR YOU

1. All information about the study comes from Keys et al., *The Biology of Human Starvation*, vols. 1 and 2.

2. Ibid., p. 810. Keys attributes it to A. W. Greely, *Three Years of Arctic Service: An Account of the Lady Franklin Bay Expedition of 1881–1884 and the Attainment of the Farthest North* (New York: Scribner, 1886).

3. Keys et al., *The Biology of Human Starvation*, vols. 1 and 2, p. 811. Keys also attributes this to Greely.

4. Ibid.

5. The man was John Franklin, and it did not end well for him the next time. Anthony Brandt, *The Man Who Ate His Boots: The Tragic History of the Search for the Northwest Passage* (New York: Knopf, 2010).

6. Keys et al., *The Biology of Human Starvation*, vols. 1 and 2, p. 776. The quote is from Keys, but he is paraphrasing a work in Czech, which I cannot access (or read): J. Stavel, *Hlad: Prispevek K Analyse Pudu* (Bratislava: Philosophy Faculty, Comenius University, 1936).

7. For this reason, some people consider the experience of these men to be more similar to the eating disorder of anorexia than to mere dieting.

8. Stephen Smith, "Battles of Belief in World War II," *American Radioworks*, 2013, http://americanradioworks.publicradio.org/features/wwii/transcript.html.

9. The exception is the set of tests that the men were trained on extensively

before starvation. They continued to do fine on those even during starvation, suggesting that you might not see impairments on well-learned processes.

10.   Michael W. Green and Nicola A. Elliman, "Are Dieting-Related Cognitive Impairments a Function of Iron Status?," *British Journal of Nutrition* 109, no. 1 (January 14, 2013): 184–92, doi:10.1017/S0007114512000864.

11.   M. W. Green et al., "Impairment of Cognitive Performance Associated with Dieting and High Levels of Dietary Restraint," *Physiology & Behavior* 55, no. 3 (March 1994): 447–52; Michael W. Green and Peter J. Rogers, "Impairments in Working Memory Associated with Spontaneous Dieting Behaviour," *Psychological Medicine* 28, no. 5 (September 1, 1998): 1063–70; Jacqueline Shaw and Marika Tiggemann, "Dieting and Working Memory: Preoccupying Cognitions and the Role of the Articulatory Control Process," *British Journal of Health Psychology* 9, Pt. 2 (May 2004): 175–85, doi:10.1348/135910704773891032; Louise Vreugdenburg, Janet Bryan, and Eva Kemps, "The Effect of Self-Initiated Weight-Loss Dieting on Working Memory: The Role of Preoccupying Cognitions," *Appetite* 41, no. 3 (2003): 291–300; P. J. Rogers and M. W. Green, "Dieting, Dietary Restraint and Cognitive Performance," *British Journal of Clinical Psychology* 32, Pt. 1 (February 1993): 113–16.

12.   Green and Rogers, "Impairments in Working Memory Associated with Spontaneous Dieting Behaviour"; Eva Kemps, Marika Tiggemann, and Kelly Marshall, "Relationship between Dieting to Lose Weight and the Functioning of the Central Executive," *Appetite* 45, no. 3 (2005): 287–94; Eva Kemps and Marika Tiggemann, "Working Memory Performance and Preoccupying Thoughts in Female Dieters: Evidence for a Selective Central Executive Impairment," *British Journal of Clinical Psychology* 44, Pt. 3 (September 2005): 357–66, doi:10.1348/014466505X35272; Vreugdenburg, Bryan, and Kemps, "The Effect of Self-Initiated Weight-Loss Dieting on Working Memory."

13.   Nicola Jones and Peter J. Rogers, "Preoccupation, Food, and Failure: An Investigation of Cognitive Performance Deficits in Dieters," *International Journal of Eating Disorders* 33, no. 2 (March 2003): 185–92, doi:10.1002/eat.10124.

14.   Michael W. Green and Peter J. Rogers, "Impaired Cognitive Functioning during Spontaneous Dieting," *Psychological Medicine* 25, no. 05 (July 9, 1995): 1003, doi:10.1017/S0033291700037491; Kemps, Tiggemann, and Marshall, "Relationship between Dieting to Lose Weight and the Functioning of the Central Executive"; Vreugdenburg, Bryan, and Kemps, "The Effect of Self-Initiated Weight-Loss Dieting on Working Memory."

15.   Vanessa Engle, quoted in Ermine Saner, "The Fat Controllers," *Guardian*, August 8, 2013.

16.   Kemps, Tiggemann, and Marshall, "Relationship between Dieting to Lose Weight and the Functioning of the Central Executive"; Kemps and Tiggemann, "Working Memory Performance and Preoccupying Thoughts in Female Dieters"; Vreugdenburg, Bryan, and Kemps, "The Effect of Self-

Initiated Weight-Loss Dieting on Working Memory."

17.   Jones and Rogers, "Preoccupation, Food, and Failure."

18.   Green and Rogers, "Impaired Cognitive Functioning during Spontaneous
       Dieting"; Kemps and Tiggemann, "Working Memory Performance and Pre-
       occupying Thoughts in Female Dieters"; Kemps, Tiggemann, and Marshall,
       "Relationship between Dieting to Lose Weight and the Functioning of the
       Central Executive"; Vreugdenburg, Bryan, and Kemps, "The Effect of Self-
       Initiated Weight-Loss Dieting on Working Memory."

19.   Green and Rogers, "Impaired Cognitive Functioning during Spontaneous
       Dieting."

20.   Hirsch, "Obesity: Matter over Mind."

21.   Kathleen D. Vohs and Brandon J. Schmeichel, "Self-Regulation and Ex-
       tended Now: Controlling the Self Alters the Subjective Experience of Time,"
       Journal of Personality and Social Psychology 85 (2003): 217–30.

22.   It's possible I am the person who said this. I've said it a lot over the years. I
       searched the Internet and can't find it at all.

23.   A. Janet Tomiyama et al., "Low Calorie Dieting Increases Cortisol,"
       Psychosomatic Medicine 72, no. 4 (May 2010): 357–64, doi:10.1097/
       PSY.0b013e3181d9523c. Also see: Michael W. Green, Nicola A. Elliman,
       and Mary J. Kretsch, "Weight Loss Strategies, Stress, and Cognitive Func-
       tion: Supervised versus Unsupervised Dieting," *Psychoneuroendocrinology* 30,
       no. 9 (2005): 908–18.

24.   Everything I say about stress in this paragraph and the next comes from Rob-
       ert Sapolsky's brilliant book, *Why Zebras Don't Get Ulcers*, 3rd ed.

25.   A. Janet Tomiyama et al., "Does Cellular Aging Relate to Patterns of Allosta-
       sis? An Examination of Basal and Stress Reactive HPA Axis Activity and
       Telomere Length," *Physiology & Behavior* 106, no. 1 (April 12, 2012): 40–45,
       doi:10.1016/j.physbeh.2011.11.016.

26.   Amy Kiefer et al., "Dietary Restraint and Telomere Length in Pre- and Post-
       Menopausal Women," *Psychosomatic Medicine* 70, no. 8 (October 1, 2008):
       845–49, doi:10.1097/PSY.0b013e318187d05e.

27.   David Gal and Wendy Liu, "Grapes of Wrath: The Angry Effects of Self-
       Control," *Journal of Consumer Research* 38, no. 3 (2011): 445–58.

28.   Keys et al., *The Biology of Human Starvation*, vols. 1 and 2, p. 907.

29.   Smith, "Battles of Belief in World War II."

30.   Thomas A. Wadden et al., "Dieting and the Development of Eating Disor-
       ders in Obese Women: Results of a Randomized Controlled Trial," *American
       Journal of Clinical Nutrition* 80, no. 3 (September 1, 2004): 560–68; Diann
       M. Ackard, Jillian K. Croll, and Ann Kearney-Cooke, "Dieting Frequency
       among College Females: Association with Disordered Eating, Body Image,
       and Related Psychological Problems," *Journal of Psychosomatic Research* 52,
       no. 3 (2002): 129–36; F. M. Cachelin and P. C. Regan, "Prevalence and
       Correlates of Chronic Dieting in a Multi-Ethnic U.S. Community Sample,"
       Eating and Weight Disorders 11, no. 2 (June 1, 2006): 91–99; Scott Crow et
       al., "Psychosocial and Behavioral Correlates of Dieting among Overweight

and Non-Overweight Adolescents," *Journal of Adolescent Health* 38, no. 5 (2006): 569–74; Meghan M. Gillen, Charlotte N. Markey, and Patrick M. Markey, "An Examination of Dieting Behaviors among Adults: Links with Depression," *Eating Behaviors* 13, no. 2 (2012): 88–93; T. A. Wadden, A. J. Stunkard, and J. W. Smoller, "Dieting and Depression: A Methodological Study," *Journal of Consulting and Clinical Psychology* 54, no. 6 (1986): 869.

31. Reviewed in Rena R. Wing et al., "Mood Changes in Behavioral Weight Loss Programs," *Journal of Psychosomatic Research* 28, no. 3 (1984): 189–96.

32. Ibid.

33. Reviewed in Jordan W. Smoller, Thomas A. Wadden, and Albert J. Stunkard, "Dieting and Depression: A Critical Review," *Journal of Psychosomatic Research* 31, no. 4 (1987): 429–40.

34. Dacher Keltner, "Evidence for the Distinctness of Embarrassment, Shame, and Guilt: A Study of Recalled Antecedents and Facial Expressions of Emotion," *Cognition & Emotion* 10, no. 2 (March 1996): 155–72, doi:10.1080/026999396380312.

35. Ben C. Fletcher et al., "How Visual Images of Chocolate Affect the Craving and Guilt of Female Dieters," *Appetite* 48, no. 2 (2007): 211–17; Gillian A. King, C. Peter Herman, and Janet Polivy, "Food Perception in Dieters and Non-Dieters," *Appetite* 8, no. 2 (1987): 147–58.

36. B. Wansink, M. Cheney, and N. Chan, "Exploring Comfort Food Preferences Across Age and Gender," *Physiology & Behavior* 79, nos. 4–5 (September 2003): 739–47, doi:10.1016/S0031-9384(03)00203-8.

37. Michael Prager, "I Don't Consider Fatness a Problem," MichaelPrager .com/blog, 2013, http://michaelprager.com/content/i-dont-consider-fatness-problem-Deb-Burgard-Health-At-Every-Size.

38. June Price Tangney, Jeff Stuewig, and Debra J Mashek, "Moral Emotions and Moral Behavior," *Annual Review of Psychology* 58 (January 2007): 345–72, doi:10.1146/annurev.psych.56.091103.070145.

39. Tara L. Gruenewald et al., "Acute Threat to the Social Self: Shame, Social Self-Esteem, and Cortisol Activity," *Psychosomatic Medicine* 66, no. 6 (January 1, 2004): 915–24, doi:10.1097/01.psy.0000143639.61693.ef.

40. Sally S. Dickerson et al., "Immunological Effects of Induced Shame and Guilt," *Psychosomatic Medicine* 66, no. 1 (2004): 124–31.

41. Tangney, Stuewig, and Mashek, "Moral Emotions and Moral Behavior."

42. Eric Stice, "Risk and Maintenance Factors for Eating Pathology: A Meta-Analytic Review," *Psychological Bulletin* 128, no. 5 (September 2002): 825–48.

43. Ibid.

44. Eric Stice et al., "Fasting Increases Risk for Onset of Binge Eating and Bulimic Pathology: A 5-Year Prospective Study," *Journal of Abnormal Psychology* 117, no. 4 (November 1, 2008): 941–46, doi:10.1037/a0013644.

45. Wadden et al., "Dieting and the Development of Eating Disorders in Obese Women."

46. Donald A. Williamson et al., "Is Caloric Restriction Associated with

Development of Eating-Disorder Symptoms? Results from the CAL-ERIE Trial," *Health Psychology* 27, no. 1 Suppl. (January 2008): S32–42, doi:10.1037/0278-6133.27.1.S32.

47.   Stice, Burger, and Yokum, "Caloric Deprivation Increases Responsivity of Attention and Reward Brain Regions to Intake, Anticipated Intake, and Images of Palatable Foods."

48.   Gene-Jack Wang et al., "Regional Brain Metabolic Activation during Craving Elicited by Recall of Previous Drug Experiences," *Life Sciences* 64, no. 9 (1999): 775–84.

49.   A. E. Field et al., "Weight Cycling, Weight Gain, and Risk of Hypertension in Women," *American Journal of Epidemiology* 150, no. 6 (1999): 573–79.

50.   Richard L. Atkinson, "Weight Cycling," *JAMA* 272, no. 15 (October 19, 1994): 1196, doi:10.1001/jama.1994.03520150064038.

51.   Mette K. Simonsen et al., "Intentional Weight Loss and Mortality among Initially Healthy Men and Women," *Nutrition Reviews* 66, no. 7 (July 2008): 375–86, doi:10.1111/j.1753-4887.2008.00047.x; M. E. Perez Morales, A. Jimenez Cruz, and M. Bacardi Gascon, "The Effect of Weight Loss on Mortality: A Systematic Review from 2000 to 2009," *Nutrición Hospitalaria* 25, no. 5 (2010): 718–24, doi:S0212-16112010000500006 [pii].

52.   M. Harrington, S. Gibson, and R. C. Cottrell, "A Review and Meta-Analysis of the Effect of Weight Loss on All-Cause Mortality Risk," *Nutrition Research Reviews* 22, no. 1 (2009): 93–108, doi:10.1017/S0954422409990035; Victoria L Stevens et al., "Weight Cycling and Mortality in a Large Prospective US Study," *American Journal of Epidemiology* 175, no. 8 (April 15, 2012): 785–92, doi:10.1093/aje/kwr378.

53.   Kelly D. Brownell and Judith Rodin, "Medical, Metabolic, and Psychological Effects of Weight Cycling," *Archives of Internal Medicine* 154, no. 12 (1994): 1325; Reubin Andres, "Long-Term Effects of Change in Body Weight on All-Cause Mortality: A Review," *Annals of Internal Medicine* 119, no. 7, Part 2 (October 1, 1993): 737, doi:10.7326/0003-4819-119-7_Part_2-199310011-00022; Perez Morales, Jimenez Cruz, and Bacardi Gascon, "The Effect of Weight Loss on Mortality: A Systematic Review from 2000 to 2009"; Simonsen et al., "Intentional Weight Loss and Mortality among Initially Healthy Men and Women."

54.   Because only 6 percent of the population is obesity class III or heavier, most people in the sample were probably obesity class I or II. It may not be the case that having a stable weight in one of the heavier obese classes is as safe. Peter Rzehak et al., "Weight Change, Weight Cycling and Mortality in the ERFORT Male Cohort Study," *European Journal of Epidemiology* 22, no. 10 (January 2007): 665–73, doi:10.1007/s10654-007-9167-5.

55.   Elizabeth Abbess, "Cabbage Soup Diet: What You Need to Know," *Discovery Fit and Health*, 2013, http://health.howstuffworks.com/wellness/diet-fitness/diets/cabbage-soup-diet2.htm.

56.   "Xenical Orlistat: Information for Consumers," 2013, http://www.xenical.com/xenical/default.do.

CHAPTER 5: OBESITY IS NOT A DEATH SENTENCE

1. Danielle Dellorto, "Obesity Bigger Health Crisis Than Hunger," CNN.com, 2012, http://edition.cnn.com/2012/12/13/health/global-burden-report/.

2. Nanci Hellmich, "Obesity on Track as No. 1 Killer," USAToday.com, March 9, 2004, http://usatoday30.usatoday.com/news/health/2004-03-09-obesity_x.htm.

3. Nanci Hellmich, "Obesity Threatens Life Expectancy," USAToday.com, 2005, http://usatoday30.usatoday.com/news/health/2005-03-16-obesity-lifespan_x.htm.

4. National Center for Health Statistics, *Health, United States, 2013: With Special Feature on Prescription Drugs* (Hyattsville, MD, 2014), Table 69.

5. S. Jay Olshansky et al., "A Potential Decline in Life Expectancy in the United States in the 21st Century," *New England Journal of Medicine* 352, no. 11 (March 17, 2005): 1138–45, doi:10.1056/NEJMsr043743.

6. N. Christenfeld, D. P. Phillips, and L. M. Glynn, "What's in a Name: Mortality and the Power of Symbols," *Journal of Psychosomatic Research* 47, no. 3 (September 1999): 241–54.

7. Katherine M. Flegal et al., "Association of All-Cause Mortality with Overweight and Obesity Using Standard Body Mass Index Categories: A Systematic Review and Meta-Analysis," *JAMA* 309, no. 1 (January 2, 2013): 71–82, doi:10.1001/jama.2012.113905.

8. These are technically hazard ratios.

9. In these paragraphs, when I say the ratio equals 1, I mean the 95 percent confidence interval around the ratio includes 1. Similarly, if I say the ratio is over 1, I mean the lower end of the 95 percent confidence interval around the ratio is greater than 1. The number 140 refers to the number of results she looked at from a total of 97 papers, not the number of papers.

10. Hazard ratio for lung cancer incidence in men who smoke a half a pack to a full pack of cigarettes per day, compared to never smokers. Neal D. Freedman et al., "Cigarette Smoking and Subsequent Risk of Lung Cancer in Men and Women: Analysis of a Prospective Cohort Study," *Lancet Oncology* 9, no. 7 (2008): 649–56.

11. Katherine M. Flegal et al., "Prevalence of Obesity and Trends in the Distribution of Body Mass Index among US Adults, 1999–2010," *JAMA* 307, no. 5 (February 1, 2012): 491–97, doi:10.1001/jama.2012.39.

12. K. M. Flegal et al., "Excess Deaths Associated with Underweight, Overweight, and Obesity," *JAMA* 293, no. 15 (2005): 1861–67, doi:10.1001/jama.293.15.1861.

13. Daphne P. Guh et al., "The Incidence of Co-Morbidities Related to Obesity and Overweight: A Systematic Review and Meta-Analysis," *BMC Public Health* 9 (January 2009): 88, doi:10.1186/1471-2458-9-88.

14. National Center for Health Statistics, *Health, United States, 2013: With Special Feature on Prescription Drugs*, Table 46.

15. Ibid., Table 44.

16. Carl J. Lavie, Richard V. Milani, and Hector O. Ventura, "Obesity and Cardiovascular Disease: Risk Factor, Paradox, and Impact of Weight Loss," *Journal of the American College of Cardiology* 53, no. 21 (May 26, 2009): 1925–32, doi:10.1016/j.jacc.2008.12.068.

17. Konstantinos Vemmos et al., "Association between Obesity and Mortality after Acute First-Ever Stroke: The Obesity-Stroke Paradox," *Stroke* 42, no. 1 (January 2011): 30–6, doi:10.1161/STROKEAHA.110.593434.

18. Mercedes R. Carnethon et al., "Association of Weight Status with Mortality in Adults with Incident Diabetes," *JAMA* 308, no. 6 (August 8, 2012): 581–90, doi:10.1001/jama.2012.9282.

19. Kamyar Kalantar-Zadeh et al., "The Obesity Paradox and Mortality Associated With Surrogates of Body Size and Muscle Mass in Patients Receiving Hemodialysis," *Mayo Clinic Proceedings* 85, no. 11 (2010): 991–1001.

20. Jordan A. Guenette, Dennis Jensen, and Denis E. O'Donnell, "Respiratory Function and the Obesity Paradox," *Current Opinion in Clinical Nutrition and Metabolic Care* 13, no. 6 (November 2010): 618–24, doi:10.1097/MCO.0b013e32833e3453.

21. Agustín Escalante, Roy W. Haas, and Inmaculada del Rincón, "Paradoxical Effect of Body Mass Index on Survival in Rheumatoid Arthritis: Role of Comorbidity and Systemic Inflammation," *Archives of Internal Medicine* 165, no. 14 (July 25, 2005): 1624–29, doi:10.1001/archinte.165.14.1624.

22. Vicente F. Corrales-Medina et al., "The Obesity Paradox in Community-Acquired Bacterial Pneumonia," *International Journal of Infectious Diseases* 15, no. 1 (2011): e54–e57.

23. Relin Yang et al., "Obesity and Weight Loss at Presentation of Lung Cancer Are Associated with Opposite Effects on Survival," *Journal of Surgical Research* 170, no. 1 (2011): e75–e83.

24. Susan Halabi et al., "Inverse Correlation between Body Mass Index and Clinical Outcomes in Men with Advanced Castration-Recurrent Prostate Cancer," *Cancer* 110, no. 7 (October 1, 2007): 1478–84, doi:10.1002/cncr.22932.

25. Henry Oliveros and Eduardo Villamor, "Obesity and Mortality in Critically Ill Adults: A Systematic Review and Meta-Analysis," *Obesity* (Silver Spring, Md.) 16, no. 3 (March 2008): 515–21, doi:10.1038/oby.2007.102; Jeptha P Curtis et al., "The Obesity Paradox: Body Mass Index and Outcomes in Patients with Heart Failure," *Archives of Internal Medicine* 165, no. 1 (January 10, 2005): 55–61, doi:10.1001/archinte.165.1.55.

26. Oliveros and Villamor, "Obesity and Mortality in Critically Ill Adults: A Systematic Review and Meta-Analysis."

27. The classic citation is: R. A. Fisher, *The Design of Experiments* (Oxford, England: Oliver & Boyd, 1935). A fantastic explanation of random assignment is in my former colleagues' textbook: Brett W. Pelham and Hart Blanton, *Conducting Research in Psychology: Measuring the Weight of Smoke*, 4th ed., (Belmont, CA: Cengage Learning, 2011). They say random assignment "is the closest thing to magic that researchers have ever discovered" (p. 202).

28. You may be thinking about the studies from Chapter 2 in which prisoners and other volunteers were made temporarily obese. Those are not useful for this purpose as they did not have control groups. Sims, "Experimental Obesity, Dietary-Induced Thermogenesis, and Their Clinical Implications."

29. Mann et al., "Medicare's Search for Effective Obesity Treatments: Diets Are Not the Answer."

30. Mann, Tomiyama, and Ahlstrom, "Long-Term Effects of Dieting."

31. Look AHEAD Research Group, "Cardiovascular Effects of Intensive Lifestyle Intervention in Type 2 Diabetes," *New England Journal of Medicine* 369, no. 2 (June 24, 2013): 145–54, doi:10.1056/NEJMoa1212914.

32. Definition appears here: National Institute of Diabetes and Digestive and Kidney Diseases, "Data & Safety Monitoring Plans," *Research and Funding for Scientists*, 2013, http://www.niddk.nih.gov/research-funding/process/human-subjects-research/data-safety-monitoring-plans/Pages/data-and-safety-monitoring-plans.aspx. Statement that Look AHEAD (see previous note) was terminated for futility appears at Look AHEAD Protocol Review Committee, "Protocol: Action for Health in Diabetes: Look AHEAD Clinical Trial, 10th Revision," 2012, https://www.lookaheadtrial.org/public/LookAHEADProtocol.pdf, p. 38.

33. "Weight Loss Does Not Lower Heart Disease Risk from Type 2 Diabetes," press release, National Institutes of Health, 2012, http://www.nih.gov/news/health/oct2012/niddk-19.htm.

34. J. Bruce Redmon et al., "Effect of the Look AHEAD Study Intervention on Medication Use and Related Cost to Treat Cardiovascular Disease Risk Factors in Individuals with Type 2 Diabetes," *Diabetes Care* 33, no. 6 (June 1, 2010): 1153–58, doi:10.2337/dc09-2090.

35. This includes all of those mortality studies that Katherine Flegal reviewed.

36. If you use random assignment, you don't have to worry about any differences there might normally be between obese and non-obese people, because random assignment makes your groups pretty much equal in pretty much every way. It even makes the groups about equal on things you never thought of. This is crucial. As a professional scientist, I can say with conviction that there is an infinite number of things I have never thought of.

37. J. J. Varo et al., "Distribution and Determinants of Sedentary Lifestyles in the European Union," *International Journal of Epidemiology* 32, no. 1 (February 1, 2003): 138–46, doi:10.1093/ije/dyg116.

38. Ibid.

39. Casazza et al., "Myths, Presumptions, and Facts about Obesity."

40. Phillipa Caudwell et al., "Exercise Alone Is Not Enough: Weight Loss Also Needs a Healthy (Mediterranean) Diet?," *Public Health Nutrition* 12, no. 9A (September 1, 2009): 1663–66, doi:10.1017/S1368980009990528.

41. Scott M. Grundy et al., "Clinical Management of Metabolic Syndrome: Report of the American Heart Association/National Heart, Lung, and Blood Institute/American Diabetes Association Conference on Scientific Issues Related to Management," *Circulation* 109, no. 4 (February 3, 2004): 551–56,

doi:10.1161/01.CIR.0000112379.88385.67.

42. D. E. Thomas, E. J. Elliott, and G. A. Naughton, "Exercise for Type 2 Diabetes Mellitus," *Evidence-Based Nursing* 10, no. 1 (2007): 11.

43. Balraj S. Heran et al., "Exercise-Based Cardiac Rehabilitation for Coronary Heart Disease," *Cochrane Database of Systematic Reviews* no. 7 (January 2011): CD001800, doi:10.1002/14651858.CD001800.pub2.

44. Paul D. Thompson et al., "Exercise and Physical Activity in the Prevention and Treatment of Atherosclerotic Cardiovascular Disease: A Statement from the Council on Clinical Cardiology (Subcommittee on Exercise, Rehabilitation, and Prevention) and the Council on Nutrition, Physical Activity, and Metabolism (Subcommittee on Physical Activity)," *Circulation* 107, no. 24 (June 24, 2003): 3109–16, doi:10.1161/01.CIR.0000075572.40158.77.

45. Sean Carroll and Mike Dudfield, "What Is the Relationship between Exercise and Metabolic Abnormalities?," *Sports Medicine* 34, no. 6 (2004): 371–418, doi:10.2165/00007256-200434060-00004.

46. Martha L. Slattery and John D. Potter, "Physical Activity and Colon Cancer: Confounding or Interaction?," *Medicine and Science in Sports and Exercise* 34, no. 6 (June 2002): 913–19.

47. Rosalind A. Breslow et al., "Long-Term Recreational Physical Activity and Breast Cancer in the National Health and Nutrition Examination Survey I Epidemiologic Follow-up Study," *Cancer Epidemiology, Biomarkers & Prevention* 10, no. 7 (July 1, 2001): 805–8.

48. Casazza et al., "Myths, Presumptions, and Facts about Obesity"; Breslow et al., "Long-Term Recreational Physical Activity and Breast Cancer in the National Health and Nutrition Examination Survey I Epidemiologic Follow-up Study"; Grundy et al., "Clinical Management of Metabolic Syndrome"; Thomas, Elliott, and Naughton, "Exercise for Type 2 Diabetes Mellitus"; Caudwell et al., "Exercise Alone Is Not Enough."

49. S. N. Blair and T. S. Church, "The Fitness, Obesity, and Health Equation: Is Physical Activity the Common Denominator?," *JAMA* 292, no. 10 (2004): 1232–34, doi:10.1001/jama.292.10.1232; S. N. Blair and S. Brodney, "Effects of Physical Inactivity and Obesity on Morbidity and Mortality: Current Evidence and Research Issues," *Medicine & Science in Sports & Exercise* 31, no. 11 Suppl. (1999): S646–62; M. Fogelholm, "Physical Activity, Fitness and Fatness: Relations to Mortality, Morbidity and Disease Risk Factors: A Systematic Review," *Obesity Reviews* 11, no. 3 (2010): 202–21, doi:10.1111/j.1467-789X.2009.00653.x; M. Wei et al., "Relationship between Low Cardiorespiratory Fitness and Mortality in Normal-Weight, Overweight, and Obese Men," *JAMA* 282, no. 16 (1999): 1547–53.

50. Paul McAuley et al., "Fitness and Fatness as Mortality Predictors in Healthy Older Men: The Veterans Exercise Testing Study," *Journals of Gerontology: Series A, Biological Sciences and Medical Sciences* 64, no. 6 (June 1, 2009): 695–99, doi:10.1093/gerona/gln039.

51. Caitlin Mason et al., "History of Weight Cycling Does Not Impede Future Weight Loss or Metabolic Improvements in Postmenopausal Women,"

Metabolism: Clinical and Experimental 62, no. 1 (January 1, 2013): 127–36, doi:10.1016/j.metabol.2012.06.012.

52. Nancy E. Adler and Joan M. Ostrove, "Socioeconomic Status and Health: What We Know and What We Don't," *Annals of the New York Academy of Sciences* 896, no. 1 (December 6, 1999): 3–15, doi:10.1111/j.1749-6632.1999. tb08101.x.

53. M. G. Marmot, M. J. Shipley, and G. Rose, "Inequalities in Death—Specific Explanations of a General Pattern?," *Lancet* 1, no. 8384 (May 5, 1984): 1003–1006.

54. Adler and Ostrove, "Socioeconomic Status and Health."

55. U.S. Department of Health and Human Services, Office of Disease Prevention and Health Promotion, *Healthy People 2020* (Washington, DC, 2010).

56. For an outstanding review, see Karen A. Matthews and Linda C. Gallo, "Psychological Perspectives on Pathways Linking Socioeconomic Status and Physical Health," *Annual Review of Psychology* 62 (January 2011): 501–30, doi:10.1146/annurev.psych.031809.130711.

57. Bruce S. McEwen and Teresa Seeman, "Protective and Damaging Effects of Mediators of Stress: Elaborating and Testing the Concepts of Allostasis and Allostatic Load," *Annals of the New York Academy of Sciences* 896, no. 1 (December 6, 1999): 30–47, doi:10.1111/j.1749-6632.1999.tb08103.x.

58. K. E. Pickett and M. Pearl, "Multilevel Analyses of Neighbourhood Socioeconomic Context and Health Outcomes: A Critical Review," *Journal of Epidemiology and Community Health* 55, no. 2 (February 2001): 111–22.

59. Youfa Wang and May A. Beydoun, "The Obesity Epidemic in the United States—Gender, Age, Socioeconomic, Racial/Ethnic, and Geographic Characteristics: A Systematic Review and Meta-Regression Analysis," *Epidemiologic Reviews* 29, no. 1 (January 1, 2007): 6–28, doi:10.1093/epirev/mxm007; J. Sobal and A. J. Stunkard, "Socioeconomic Status and Obesity: A Review of the Literature," *Psychological Bulletin* 105, no. 2 (1989): 260–75.

60. Jacob J. Feldman et al., "National Trends in Educational Differentials in Mortality," *American Journal of Epidemiology* 129, no. 5 (May 1, 1989): 919–33; M. G. Marmot et al., "Health Inequalities among British Civil Servants: The Whitehall II Study," *Lancet* 337, no. 8754 (June 8, 1991): 1387–93; Marmot, Shipley, and Rose, "Inequalities in Death—Specific Explanations of a General Pattern?"; H. Bosma et al., "Low Control Beliefs, Classical Coronary Risk Factors, and Socio-Economic Differences in Heart Disease in Older Persons," *Social Science & Medicine* 60, no. 4 (2005): 737–45.

61. National Institutes of Health, U.S. Department of Health and Human Services, "What Is Metabolic Syndrome?," *Health Information for the Public*, accessed November 5, 2013, http://www.nhlbi.nih.gov/health/health-topics/topics/ms/.

62. Thais Coutinho et al., "Combining Body Mass Index with Measures of Central Obesity in the Assessment of Mortality in Subjects with Coronary Disease: Role of 'Normal Weight Central Obesity,'" *Journal of the American*

College of Cardiology 61, no. 5 (February 5, 2013): 553–60, doi:10.1016/j.jacc.2012.10.035; Thais Coutinho et al., "Central Obesity and Survival in Subjects with Coronary Artery Disease: A Systematic Review of the Literature and Collaborative Analysis with Individual Subject Data," *Journal of the American College of Cardiology* 57, no. 19 (May 10, 2011): 1877–86, doi:10.1016/j.jacc.2010.11.058; Halfdan Petursson et al., "Body Configuration as a Predictor of Mortality: Comparison of Five Anthropometric Measures in a 12 Year Follow-up of the Norwegian HUNT 2 Study," ed. Stefan Kiechl, *PloS One* 6, no. 10 (January 2011): e26621, doi:10.1371/journal.pone.0026621.

63.   Coutinho et al., "Central Obesity and Survival in Subjects with Coronary Artery Disease."

64.   Elizabeth A. Pascoe and Laura Smart Richman, "Perceived Discrimination and Health: A Meta-Analytic Review," *Psychological Bulletin* 135, no. 4 (2009): 531–54.

65.   R. M. Puhl and C. A. Heuer, "The Stigma of Obesity: A Review and Update," *Obesity* (Silver Spring, MD) 17, no. 5 (2009): 941–64, doi:10.1038/oby.2008.636.

66.   Drew A. Anderson and Thomas A. Wadden, "Bariatric Surgery Patients' Views of Their Physicians' Weight-Related Attitudes and Practices," *Obesity Research* 12, no. 10 (October 2004): 1587–95, doi:10.1038/oby.2004.198.

67.   Rebecca M. Puhl and Kelly D. Brownell, "Confronting and Coping with Weight Stigma: An Investigation of Overweight and Obese Adults," *Obesity* (Silver Spring, MD) 14, no. 10 (October 2006): 1802–15, doi:10.1038/oby.2006.208.

68.   N. K. Amy et al., "Barriers to Routine Gynecological Cancer Screening for White and African-American Obese Women," *International Journal of Obesity* 30, no. 1 (January 4, 2006): 147–55, doi:10.1038/sj.ijo.0803105.

69.   G. D. Foster et al., "Primary Care Physicians' Attitudes about Obesity and Its Treatment," *Obesity Research* 11, no. 10 (2003): 1168–77, doi:10.1038/oby.2003.161.

70.   M. B. Schwartz et al., "Weight Bias among Health Professionals Specializing in Obesity," *Obesity Research* 11, no. 9 (2003): 1033–39.

71.   M. R. Hebl and J. Xu, "Weighing the Care: Physicians' Reactions to the Size of a Patient," *International Journal of Obesity and Related Metabolic Disorders* 25, no. 8 (August 2001): 1246–52, doi:10.1038/sj.ijo.0801681.

72.   Kimberly A. Gudzune et al., "Physicians Build Less Rapport with Obese Patients," *Obesity* (Silver Spring, MD) 21, no. 10 (March 20, 2013): 2146–52, doi:10.1002/oby.20384.

73.   David P. Miller et al., "Are Medical Students Aware of Their Anti-Obesity Bias?," *Academic Medicine* 88, no. 7 (July 2013): 978–82, doi:10.1097/ACM.0b013e318294f817; Sean M. Phelan et al., "Implicit and Explicit Weight Bias in a National Sample of 4,732 Medical Students: The Medical Student CHANGES Study," *Obesity* (Silver Spring, MD) (2013), doi:10.1002/oby.20687.

74. Kimberly A. Gudzune et al., "Doctor Shopping by Overweight and Obese Patients Is Associated with Increased Healthcare Utilization," *Obesity* (Silver Spring, MD) 21, no. 7 (July 2013): 1328–34, doi:10.1002/oby.20189.

75. T. Ostbye et al., "Associations between Obesity and Receipt of Screening Mammography, Papanicolaou Tests, and Influenza Vaccination: Results from the Health and Retirement Study (HRS) and the Asset and Health Dynamics among the Oldest Old (AHEAD) Study," *American Journal of Public Health* 95, no. 9 (2005): 1623–30, doi:10.2105/AJPH.2004.047803; C. C. Wee et al., "Screening for Cervical and Breast Cancer: Is Obesity an Unrecognized Barrier to Preventive Care?," *Annals of Internal Medicine* 132, no. 9 (2000): 697–704.

76. Ostbye et al., "Associations between Obesity and Receipt of Screening Mammography, Papanicolaou Tests, and Influenza Vaccination"; Wee et al., "Screening for Cervical and Breast Cancer."

77. Jeanne M. Ferrante et al., "Colorectal Cancer Screening among Obese Versus Non-Obese Patients in Primary Care Practices," *Cancer Detection and Prevention* 30, no. 5 (2006): 459–65; Allison B. Rosen and Eric C. Schneider, "Colorectal Cancer Screening Disparities Related to Obesity and Gender," *Journal of General Internal Medicine* 19, no. 4 (April 2004): 332–38, doi:10.1111/j.1525-1497.2004.30339.x.

78. Ostbye et al., "Associations between Obesity and Receipt of Screening Mammography, Papanicolaou Tests, and Influenza Vaccination."

79. Pascoe and Richman, "Perceived Discrimination and Health."

80. B. Major, D. Eliezer, and H. Rieck, "The Psychological Weight of Weight Stigma," *Social Psychological and Personality Science* 3, no. 6 (January 19, 2012): 651–58, doi:10.1177/1948550611434400. Also see Janet Tomiyama et al., "Associations of Weight Stigma with Cortisol and Oxidative Stress Independent of Adiposity," *Health Psychology* 33, no. 8 (August 2014): 862–67, doi:10.1037/hea0000107. Another example appears in Natasha A. Schvey, Rebecca M. Puhl, and Kelly D. Brownell, "The Stress of Stigma: Exploring the Effect of Weight Stigma on Cortisol Reactivity," *Psychosomatic Medicine* (2014): PSY–0000000000000031.

81. Puhl and Brownell, "Confronting and Coping with Weight Stigma."

82. Jenny H. Ledikwe et al., "Dietary Energy Density Is Associated with Energy Intake and Weight Status in US Adults," *American Journal of Clinical Nutrition* 83, no. 6 (June 2006): 1362–68.

83. Lawrence de Koning et al., "Sugar-Sweetened and Artificially Sweetened Beverage Consumption and Risk of Type 2 Diabetes in Men," *American Journal of Clinical Nutrition* 93, no. 6 (June 1, 2011): 1321–27, doi:10.3945/ajcn.110.007922. koning.

84. Ankur Vyas et al., "Diet Drink Consumption and the Risk of Cardiovascular Events: A Report from the Women's Health Initiative," *Journal of the American College of Cardiology* 63, no. 12 (April 1, 2014): A1290, doi:10.1016/S0735-1097(14)61290-0. vyas.

85. Jotham Suez et al., "Artificial Sweeteners Induce Glucose Intolerance by

Altering the Gut Microbiota," *Nature* (September 17, 2014), doi:10.1038/
nature13793. suez.

86.   A. S. Levy and A. W. Heaton, "Weight Control Practices of US Adults Try-
      ing to Lose Weight," *Annals of Internal Medicine* 119, no. 7 Part 2 (1993):
      661–66; Edward C. Weiss et al., "Weight-Control Practices among U.S.
      Adults, 2001–2002," *American Journal of Preventive Medicine* 31, no. 1
      (2006): 18–24.

87.   Lisa L. Ioannides-Demos et al., "Safety of Drug Therapies Used for Weight
      Loss and Treatment of Obesity," *Drug Safety* 29, no. 4 (2006): 277–302,
      doi:10.2165/00002018-200629040-00001.

88.   M. A. Whisman, "Loneliness and the Metabolic Syndrome in a Population-
      Based Sample of Middle-Aged and Older Adults," *Health Psychology* 29, no.
      5 (2010): 550–54, doi:10.1037/a0020760.

89.   J. Holt-Lunstad, T. B. Smith, and J. B. Layton, "Social Relationships and
      Mortality Risk: A Meta-Analytic Review," *PLoS Med* 7, no. 7 (2010):
      e1000316, doi:10.1371/journal.pmed.1000316.

90.   These came from the online supplemental materials to the article. They don't
      have a freestanding URL of their own, but can be reached from the main
      article: Flegal et al., "Association of All-Cause Mortality with Overweight
      and Obesity Using Standard Body Mass Index Categories."

91.   They had to do so by measuring at least two of the three components (for
      example, education and income) of SES, according to P. A. Braveman et
      al., "Socioeconomic Status in Health Research: One Size Does Not Fit All,"
      JAMA 294, no. 22 (2005): 2879–88, doi:10.1001/jama.294.22.2879.

92.   I reported the number for white people who had never smoked. Eric A.
      Finkelstein et al., "Individual and Aggregate Years-of-Life-Lost Associated
      with Overweight and Obesity," *Obesity* 18, no. 2 (February 2010): 333–39,
      doi:10.1038/oby.2009.253.

93.   Ibid.

94.   Christenfeld, Phillips, and Glynn, "What's in a Name."

95.   P. Campos et al., "The Epidemiology of Overweight and Obesity: Public
      Health Crisis or Moral Panic?," *International Journal of Epidemiology* 35, no.
      1 (2006): 55–60, doi:10.1093/ije/dyi254.

96.   Davidoff, "Sponsorship, Authorship, and Accountability."

97.   Olshansky et al., "A Potential Decline in Life Expectancy in the United
      States in the 21st Century."

98.   W. Wayt Gibbs, "Obesity: An Overblown Epidemic?," *Scientific American*
      292, no. 6 (June 2005): 70–77, doi:10.1038/scientificamerican0605-70.

99.   Olshansky et al., "A Potential Decline in Life Expectancy in the United
      States in the 21st Century"; David Allison, "Disclosure of Financial Infor-
      mation," *New England Journal of Medicine*, 2005, http://www.nejm.org/doi/
      suppl/10.1056/NEJMsr043743/suppl_file/1138sa1.pdf.

100. Flegal et al., "Association of All-Cause Mortality with Overweight and Obe-
      sity Using Standard Body Mass Index Categories."

CHAPTER 6: LESSONS FROM A LEAN PIG

1. I have changed his name at his request.

2. Walter Mischel, "From Good Intentions to Willpower," in *The Psychology of Action: Linking Cognition and Motivation to Behavior*, ed. Peter Gollwitzer and John Bargh (New York: Guilford Press, 1996), 197–218.

3. We cover this strategy (and many others) in our review of self-control strategies: Traci Mann, Denise de Ridder, and Kentaro Fujita, "Self-Regulation of Health Behavior: Social Psychological Approaches to Goal Setting and Goal Striving," *Health Psychology* 32, no. 5 (May 2013): 487–98, doi:10.1037/a0028533.

4. Lisa R. Young and Marion Nestle, "The Contribution of Expanding Portion Sizes to the US Obesity Epidemic," *American Journal of Public Health* 92, no. 2 (February 1, 2002): 246–49.

5. Ibid.

6. Nancy Rivera, "Ice Cream Firm Turns 40: Baskin-Robbins Starts Program to Revitalize," *Los Angeles Times*, May 6, 1985.

7. Young and Nestle, "The Contribution of Expanding Portion Sizes to the US Obesity Epidemic."

8. Ibid.

9. B. Wansink and C. S. Wansink, "The Largest Last Supper: Depictions of Food Portions and Plate Size Increased Over the Millennium," *International Journal of Obesity* (2005) 34, no. 5 (May 2010): 943–4, doi:10.1038/ijo.2010.37.

10. Ibid.

11. For a review, see Brian Wansink, "Environmental Factors That Increase the Food Intake and Consumption Volume of Unknowing Consumers," *Annual Review of Nutrition* 24 (January 2004): 455–79, doi:10.1146/annurev.nutr.24.012003.132140. Also see Carmen Piernas and Barry M. Popkin, "Increased Portion Sizes from Energy-Dense Foods Affect Total Energy Intake at Eating Occasions in US Children and Adolescents: Patterns and Trends by Age Group and Sociodemographic Characteristics, 1977–2006," *American Journal of Clinical Nutrition* 94, no. 5 (November 1, 2011): 1324–32, doi:10.3945/ajcn.110.008466; David A. Levitsky and Trisha Youn, "The More Food Young Adults Are Served, the More They Overeat," *Journal of Nutrition* 134, no. 10 (October 1, 2004): 2546–49.

12. Brian Wansink, "Can Package Size Accelerate Usage Volume?," *Journal of Marketing* 60, no. 3 (1996): 1–14, doi:10.2307/1251838.

13. Brian Wansink, Koert van Ittersum, and James E. Painter, "Ice Cream Illusions: Bowls, Spoons, and Self-Served Portion Sizes," *American Journal of Preventive Medicine* 31, no. 3 (2006): 240–43.

14. Ellen van Kleef, Christos Kavvouris, and Hans C. M. van Trijp, "The Unit Size Effect of Indulgent Food: How Eating Smaller Sized Items Signals Impulsivity and Makes Consumers Eat Less," *Psychology & Health* 29, no. 9 (September 2014): 1081–1103, doi:10.1080/08870446.2014.909426.

15.   Brian Wansink, James E. Painter, and Jill North, "Bottomless Bowls: Why Visual Cues of Portion Size May Influence Intake," *Obesity Research* 13, no. 1 (January 2005): 93–100, doi:10.1038/oby.2005.12.

16.   Ibid.

17.   B. Wansink and K. Van Ittersum, "Illusive Consumption Behavior and the DelBoeuf Illusion: Are the Eyes Really Bigger than the Stomach?," *Annual Review of Nutrition* 24 (2004): 455–79.

18.   Wansink, Painter, and North, "Bottomless Bowls."

19.   Piernas and Popkin, "Increased Portion Sizes from Energy-Dense Foods Affect Total Energy Intake at Eating Occasions in US Children and Adolescents."

20.   Frank McIntyre, "U.S. Companies Shrink Packages as Food Prices Rise," *Daily Finance*, 2011, http://www.dailyfinance.com/2011/04/04/u-s-companies-shrink-packages-as-food-prices-rise/.

21.   "Saving on Toilet Paper," OccupiedLife.com, 2011, http://occupiedlife.com/saving-on-toilet-paper/; Peggy Wang, "46 Penny-Pinching Ways to Save a Lot of Money This Year," Buzzfeed.com, 2013, http://www.buzzfeed.com/peggy/46-penny-pinching-ways-to-save-a-lot-of-money-this.

22.   Keith Hawton et al., "Long Term Effect of Reduced Pack Sizes of Paracetamol on Poisoning Deaths and Liver Transplant Activity in England and Wales: Interrupted Time Series Analyses," *BMJ (Clinical Research Ed.)* 346 (January 2013): f403; K. Hawton, "Effects of Legislation Restricting Pack Sizes of Paracetamol and Salicylate on Self Poisoning in the United Kingdom: Before and After Study," *BMJ* 322, no. 7296 (May 19, 2001): 1203, doi:10.1136/bmj.322.7296.1203.

23.   Josje Maas et al., "Do Distant Foods Decrease Intake? The Effect of Food Accessibility on Consumption," *Psychology & Health* 27, Suppl. 2 (October 2012): 59–73, doi:10.1080/08870446.2011.565341. Also see Gregory J. Privitera and Faris M. Zuraikat, "Proximity of Foods in a Competitive Food Environment Influences Consumption of a Low Calorie and a High Calorie Food," *Appetite* 76 (May 2014): 175–79, doi:10.1016/j.appet.2014.02.004.

24.   Maas et al., "Do Distant Foods Decrease Intake?"

25.   Paul Rozin et al., "Nudge to Nobesity I: Minor Changes in Accessibility Decrease Food Intake," *Judgment and Decision Making* 6, no. 4 (2011): 323–32.

26.   As far as I can tell, nobody's done this study, so this is just a speculation.

27.   For example, Frances Martel, "Jon Stewart Rails Against Bloomberg's 'Draconian' Soda Ban with Piles of Gross 'Legal' Food," Mediaite.com, 2012, http://www.mediaite.com/tv/jon-stewart-rails-against-bloombergs-draconian-soda-ban-with-piles-of-gross-legal-food/.

28.   Cecilia Kang, "Google Crunches Data on Munching in Office," *Washington Post*, September 1, 2013. Also see B. Wansink, J. E. Painter, and Y. K. Lee, "The Office Candy Dish: Proximity's Influence on Estimated and Actual Consumption," *International Journal of Obesity* 30, no. 5 (May 17, 2006): 871–75, doi:10.1038/sj.ijo.0803217; James E. Painter, Brian Wansink, and Julie B. Hieggelke, "How Visibility and Convenience Influence

Candy Consumption," *Appetite* 38, no. 3 (June 2002): 237–38, doi:10.1006/appe.2002.0485.

29. Carol E. Cornell, Judith Rodin, and Harvey Weingarten, "Stimulus-Induced Eating When Satiated," *Physiology & Behavior* 45, no. 4 (1989): 695–704.

30. If you want to be inspired to attempt it, the chef and writer Tamar Adler has posted a video online that shows her washing and roasting a huge amount of vegetables at once, which she then puts in jars in her fridge to eat on their own or use in recipes during the week. (It's a lot more exciting than it sounds.) Tamar E. Adler, "How to Stride Ahead: Part 2," Tamareadler.com, 2011, http://www.tamareadler.com/2011/10/10/how-to-stride-ahead-part-2/.

31. Joe Redden, Zata Vickers, Marla Reicks, and Elton Mykerezi, along with graduate students Stephanie Elsbernd and Nikki Miller.

32. All of the tests appear in Joseph P. Redden et al., "The Effect of Juxtaposition on the Intake of Healthy Foods" (n.d.).

CHAPTER 7: HOW TO TRICK YOUR FRIENDS INTO IGNORING A COOKIE

1.   Solomon E. Asch, "Studies of Independence and Conformity: I. A Minority of One against a Unanimous Majority," *Psychological Monographs: General and Applied*" 70, no. 9 (1956) 1–70.

2.   This effect has been replicated over 100 times across 17 countries. For a review, see Rod Bond and Peter B. Smith, "Culture and Conformity: A Meta-Analysis of Studies Using Asch's (1952b, 1956) Line Judgment Task," *Psychological Bulletin* 119, no. 1 (1996): 111–37.

3.   M. Sherif, *The Psychology of Social Norms* (Oxford, England: Harper, 1936).

4.   Paul Rozin, "The Integration of Biological, Social, Cultural and Psychological Influences on Food Choice," in *The Psychology of Food Choice*, ed. Richard Shepherd and Monique Raats (Oxfordshire, England: CABI, 2006), 19–40.

5.   John M. de Castro and E. Marie Brewer, "The Amount Eaten in Meals by Humans Is a Power Function of the Number of People Present," *Physiology & Behavior* 51, no. 1 (1992): 121–25.

6.   Ibid.; A. Ward and T. Mann, "Don't Mind If I Do: Disinhibited Eating Under Cognitive Load," *Journal of Personality and Social Psychology* 78, no. 4 (April 2000): 753–63.

7.   Vanessa I. Clendenen, C. Peter Herman, and Janet Polivy, "Social Facilitation of Eating among Friends and Strangers," *Appetite* 23, no. 1 (1994): 1–13; Sarah-Jeanne Salvy et al., "Effects of Social Influence on Eating in Couples, Friends and Strangers," *Appetite* 49, no. 1 (July 2007): 92–99, doi:10.1016/j.appet.2006.12.004.

8.   de Castro and Brewer, "The Amount Eaten in Meals by Humans Is a Power Function of the Number of People Present."

9.   Maryhope Howland, Jeffrey M. Hunger, and Traci Mann, "Friends Don't Let Friends Eat Cookies: Effects of Restrictive Eating Norms on Consumption among Friends," *Appetite* 59, no. 2 (October 2012): 505–9, doi:10.1016/

j.appet.2012.06.020. The day after our paper came out an article was published saying that people don't take research findings seriously if they come from a paper with a silly title. Uh-oh.

10.   Leon Festinger, "A Theory of Social Comparison Processes," *Human Relations* 7, no. 2 (1954): 117–40.

11.   Noah J. Goldstein, Robert B. Cialdini, and Vladas Griskevicius, "A Room with a Viewpoint: Using Social Norms to Motivate Environmental Conservation in Hotels," *Journal of Consumer Research* 35, no. 3 (October 3, 2008): 472–82, doi:10.1086/586910.

12.   Other factors matter, too, including convenience and effort, but these are equated in many countries and you still see these differences. Eric J. Johnson and Daniel Goldstein, "Do Defaults Save Lives?," *Science* 302, no. 5649 (November 21, 2003): 1338–39, doi:10.1126/science.1091721.

13.   Ervin Staub, "Instigation to Goodness: The Role of Social Norms and Interpersonal Influence," *Journal of Social Issues* 28, no. 3 (July 1972): 131–50, doi:10.1111/j.1540-4560.1972.tb00036.x.

14.   Howland, Hunger, and Mann, "Friends Don't Let Friends Eat Cookies." Other studies also show the effect of implied norms on eating, for example, Eric Robinson, Helen Benwell, and Suzanne Higgs, "Food Intake Norms Increase and Decrease Snack Food Intake in a Remote Confederate Study," *Appetite* 65 (2013): 20–24. For a review, see Eric Robinson et al., "What Everyone Else Is Eating: A Systematic Review and Meta-Analysis of the Effect of Informational Eating Norms on Eating Behavior," *Journal of the Academy of Nutrition and Dietetics* 114, no. 3 (2013): 414–29.

15.   F. Marijn Stok et al., "Minority Talks: The Influence of Descriptive Social Norms on Fruit Intake," *Psychology & Health* 27, no. 8 (January 2012): 956–70, doi:10.1080/08870446.2011.635303.

16.   Clayton Neighbors, Mary E. Larimer, and Melissa A. Lewis, "Targeting Misperceptions of Descriptive Drinking Norms: Efficacy of a Computer-Delivered Personalized Normative Feedback Intervention," *Journal of Consulting and Clinical Psychology* 72, no. 3 (June 2004): 434–47, doi:10.1037/0022-006X.72.3.434.

17.   Elizabeth M. Condon, Mary Kay Crepinsek, and Mary Kay Fox, "School Meals: Types of Foods Offered to and Consumed by Children at Lunch and Breakfast," *Journal of the American Dietetic Association* 109, no. 2 (2009): S67–S78.

18.   I worked on this with my University of Minnesota colleagues Marla Reicks, Zata Vickers, Joe Redden, and Elton Mykerezi. Marla Reicks et al., "Photographs in Lunch Tray Compartments and Vegetable Consumption among Children in Elementary School Cafeterias," *JAMA* 307, no. 8 (February 22, 2012): 784–85, doi:10.1001/jama.2012.170.

19.   Ibid.

20.   A classic finding in cognitive psychology is that people cannot remember which elements go where on a penny. Raymond S. Nickerson and Marilyn Jager Adams, "Long-Term Memory for a Common Object," *Cognitive*

Psychology 11, no. 3 (1979): 287–307.

21. Heather Barry Kappes and Patrick E. Shrout, "When Goal Sharing Produces Support That Is Not Caring," *Personality & Social Psychology Bulletin* 37, no. 5 (May 1, 2011): 662–73, doi:10.1177/0146167211399926.

22. Mary Ann Parris Stephens et al., "Spouses' Attempts to Regulate Day-to-Day Dietary Adherence among Patients with Type 2 Diabetes," *Health Psychology* 32, no. 10 (October 2013): 1029–37, doi:10.1037/a0030018; J. S. Tucker and J. S. Mueller, "Spouses' Social Control of Health Behaviors: Use and Effectiveness of Specific Strategies," *Personality and Social Psychology Bulletin* 26, no. 9 (November 1, 2000): 1120–30, doi:10.1177/01461672002611008.

23. Ibid.

24. Maryhope Howland and Jeffry A. Simpson, "Getting in Under the Radar. A Dyadic View of Invisible Support," *Psychological Science* 21, no. 12 (December 1, 2010): 1878–85, doi:10.1177/0956797610388817.

25. Marci E. J. Gleason et al., "Daily Supportive Equity in Close Relationships," *Personality & Social Psychology Bulletin* 29, no. 8 (August 1, 2003): 1036–45, doi:10.1177/0146167203253473.

CHAPTER 8: DON'T CALL THAT APPLE HEALTHY

1. The classic work on this in social psychology is in Lee Ross and Richard E. Nisbett, *The Person and the Situation* (New York: McGraw-Hill, 1991). Cognitive-behavioral therapy has a similar conceptual backbone, and is summarized nicely in David D. Burns, *Feeling Good: The New Mood Therapy*, rev. ed. (New York: William Morrow Paperbacks, 1999).

2. Brian Wansink, Koert van Ittersum, and James E. Painter, "How Descriptive Food Names Bias Sensory Perceptions in Restaurants," *Food Quality and Preference* 16, no. 5 (2005): 393–400.

3. Alia J. Crum et al., "Mind Over Milkshakes: Mindsets, Not Just Nutrients, Determine Ghrelin Response," *Health Psychology* 30, no. 4 (2011): 424–29.

4. Ibid.

5. Calorie information is per slice, six slices per pie. "Bakers Square Restaurant and Bakery Nutritional Information," Bakerssquare.com, accessed February 7, 2014, http://www.bakerssquare.com/files/nutrition.pdf.

6. H.R. 3590, 111th Congress: Patient Protection and Affordable Care Act. Public Law No. 111-148, www.GovTrack.us, 2010.

7. Kamila M Kiszko et al., "The Influence of Calorie Labeling on Food Orders and Consumption: A Review of the Literature," *Journal of Community Health* (April 24, 2014), doi:10.1007/s10900-014-9876-0. Also see Table 2 in: J. Krieger and B. E. Saelens, *Impact of Menu Labeling on Consumer Behavior: A 2008–2012 Update* (Minneapolis, MN, 2013).

8. Brian Elbel et al., "Calorie Labeling, Fast Food Purchasing and Restaurant Visits," *Obesity* (Silver Spring, MD) (October 17, 2013), doi:10.1002/oby.20550.

9. Sarah Campos, Juliana Doxey, and David Hammond, "Nutrition Labels on Pre-Packaged Foods: A Systematic Review," *Public Health Nutrition* 14, no. 8 (2011): 1496; Klaus G. Grunert and Josephine M. Wills, "A Review of European Research on Consumer Response to Nutrition Information on Food Labels," *Journal of Public Health* 15, no. 5 (April 14, 2007): 385–99, doi:10.1007/s10389-007-0101-9; Gill Cowburn and Lynn Stockley, "Consumer Understanding and Use of Nutrition Labelling: A Systematic Review," *Public Health Nutrition* 8, no. 1 (February 2005): 21–28.

10. Grunert and Wills, "A Review of European Research on Consumer Response to Nutrition Information on Food Labels"; Cowburn and Stockley, "Consumer Understanding and Use of Nutrition Labelling."

11. E. A. Wartella et al., *Front-of-Package Nutrition Rating Systems and Symbols: Promoting Healthier Choices: Phase II Report* (Washington, DC: National Academies Press, Institute of Medicine, 2011).

12. American Heart Association, "Heart Check Food Certification Program," 2014, http://www.heart.org/HEARTORG/GettingHealthy/NutritionCenter/HeartSmartShopping/Heart-Check-Program_UCM_300133_Article.jsp.

13. Christina A. Roberto et al., "Facts Up Front Versus Traffic Light Food Labels: A Randomized Controlled Trial," *American Journal of Preventive Medicine* 43, no. 2 (August 1, 2012): 134–41, doi:10.1016/j.amepre.2012.04.022.

14. We call it a check mark. "Heart Foundation Tick," Heart Foundation New Zealand, 2014, http://www.heartfoundation.org.nz/healthy-living/healthy-eating/heart-foundation-tick.

15. Ellis L. Vyth et al., "A Front-of-Pack Nutrition Logo: A Quantitative and Qualitative Process Evaluation in the Netherlands," *Journal of Health Communication* 14, no. 7 (January 2009): 631–45, doi:10.1080/10810730903204247; Gray Nathan, "Healthy Logo: Netherlands 'Choices' Logo Confirmed as First Government-Backed Scheme in EU," FoodNavigator.com, 2016, http://www.foodnavigator.com/Legislation/Healthy-logo-Netherlands-Choices-logo-confirmed-as-first-government-backed-scheme-in-EU.

16. Wartella et al., *Front-of-Package Nutrition Rating Systems and Symbols*; Roberto et al., "Facts Up Front Versus Traffic Light Food Labels."

17. Kelly D. Brownell and Jeffrey P. Koplan, "Front-of-Package Nutrition Labeling—An Abuse of Trust by the Food Industry?," *New England Journal of Medicine* 364, no. 25 (June 22, 2011): 2373–75, doi:10.1056/NEJMp1101033.

18. It was originally called Nutrition Keys. "GMA and FMI Select Agency Partners to Support $50 Million Nutrition Keys Consumer Education Campaign," FactsUpFront.org, 2011, http://www.factsupfront.org/Newsroom/5.

19. Brownell and Koplan, "Front-of-Package Nutrition Labeling."

20. Roberto et al., "Facts Up Front Versus Traffic Light Food Labels."

21. At least in the United States. Rajagopal Raghunathan, Rebecca Walker Naylor, and Wayne D. Hoyer, "The Unhealthy=Tasty Intuition and Its Effects on Taste Inferences, Enjoyment, and Choice of Food Products," *Journal of Marketing* 70 (2006): 170–84. But this may not be true in France.

Carolina O. C. Werle, Olivier Trendel, and Gauthier Ardito, "Unhealthy Food Is Not Tastier for Everybody: The 'Healthy=Tasty' French Intuition," *Food Quality and Preference* 28, no. 1 (April 2013): 116–21, doi:10.1016/j.foodqual.2012.07.007.

22.   Stacey R. Finkelstein and Ayelet Fishbach, "When Healthy Food Makes You Hungry," *Journal of Consumer Research* 37, no. 3 (October 2010): 357–67, doi:10.1086/652248.

23.   My colleagues were not aware that my lab was collecting data on these foods at the conference. They are in no way complicit in my deception.

24.   American Heart Association, "Heart Check Food Certification Program."

25.   Richard E. Nisbett and Timothy D. Wilson, "Telling More Than We Can Know: Verbal Reports on Mental Processes," *Psychological Review* 84, no. 3 (1977): 231–59.

26.   Heather Scherschel Wagner, Maryhope Howland, and Traci Mann, "Effects of Subtle and Explicit Health Messages on Food Choice," *Health Psychology*, 2014, doi:10.1037/hea0000045.

27.   Sharon S. Brehm and Jack Williams Brehm, *Psychological Reactance: A Theory of Freedom and Control* (New York: Academic Press, 1981).

28.   Including future honors student Hallie Espel and future lab manager Britt Ahlstrom.

29.   Maryhope Howland and my lab manager Toni Gabrieli.

30.   Theresa Marteau and her lab at the University of Cambridge have also shown that the word "healthy" does not lead more people to take apples, although "healthy and succulent" does. Suzanna E. Forwood et al., "Choosing between an Apple and a Chocolate Bar: The Impact of Health and Taste Labels," ed. Sidney Arthur Simon, *PloS One* 8, no. 10 (January 2013): e77500, doi:10.1371/journal.pone.0077500.

31.   Finkelstein and Fishbach, "When Healthy Food Makes You Hungry."

32.   This study is a little tricky. Both sandwiches are unhealthy, but participants believe the Big Mac is unhealthy and the Subway sandwich is healthy. P. Chandon and Brian Wansink, "The Biasing Health Halos of Fast Food Restaurant Health Claims: Lower Calorie Estimates and Higher Side Dish Consumption Intentions," *Journal of Consumer Research* 34, no. October (2007): 301–14.

33.   It's a brilliant and hugely influential study. I've never taught a course on eating, health psychology, or research methods without discussing it. Herman and Mack, "Restrained and Unrestrained Eating."

34.   Janet Polivy and C. Peter Herman, "Dieting and Binging: A Causal Analysis," *American Psychologist* 40, no. 2 (1985): 193–201.

35.   Janet Tomiyama and Ashley Moskovich.

36.   Janet Tomiyama et al., "Consumption after a Diet Violation: Disinhibition or Compensation?," *Psychological Science* 20, no. 10 (October 2009): 1275–81, doi:10.1111/j.1467-9280.2009.02436.x.

37.   Ravi Dhar and Itamar Simonson, "Making Complementary Choices in Consumption Episodes: Highlighting Versus Balancing," *Journal of Marketing Research* (1999): 29–44.

38. Kentaro Fujita et al., "Construal Levels and Self-Control," *Journal of Person-ality and Social Psychology* 90, no. 3 (March 2006): 351–67, doi:10.1037/002 2-3514.90.3.351.

39. Tinuke Oluyomi Daniel, Christina M Stanton, and Leonard H. Epstein, "The Future Is Now: Reducing Impulsivity and Energy Intake Using Epi-sodic Future Thinking," *Psychological Science* 24, no. 11 (November 1, 2013): 2339–42, doi:10.1177/0956797613488780.

40. K. Fujita and J. J. Carnevale, "Transcending Temptation Through Ab-straction: The Role of Construal Level in Self-Control," *Current Di-rections in Psychological Science* 21, no. 4 (July 25, 2012): 248–52, doi:10.1177/0963721412449169.

41. Wansink, van Ittersum, and Painter, "How Descriptive Food Names Bias Sensory Perceptions in Restaurants."

42. Walter Mischel and Nancy Baker, "Cognitive Appraisals and Transforma-tions in Delay Behavior," *Journal of Personality and Social Psychology* 31, no. 2 (1975): 254.

43. Remember when I said only one out of three hundred social psychologists at the conference figured out we were doing an experiment on them (with the apples)? That would be Ken Fujita. You can't get anything past him.

44. Kentaro Fujita and H. Anna Han, "Moving Beyond Deliberative Control of Impulses: The Effect of Construal Levels on Evaluative Associations in Self-Control Conflicts," *Psychological Science* 20, no. 7 (July 1, 2009): 799–804, doi:10.1111/j.1467-9280.2009.02372.x; Kentaro Fujita, "Seeing the Forest Beyond the Trees: A Construal-Level Approach to Self-Control," *Social and Personality Psychology Compass* 2, no. 3 (May 2008): 1475–96, doi:10.1111/ j.1751-9004.2008.00118.x.

45. Fujita and Han, "Moving Beyond Deliberative Control of Impulses."

CHAPTER 9: KNOW WHEN TO TURN OFF YOUR BRAIN

1. Jon Henley, "Merde Most Foul," *Guardian*, April 12, 2002, http://www .theguardian.com/world/2002/apr/12/worlddispatch.jonhenley.

2. Suzanne Daley, "Budget Cuts May Foul Sidewalks of Paris," *New York Times*, November 6, 2001, http://www.nytimes.com/2001/11/06/world/budget-cuts-may-foul-sidewalks-of-paris.html.

3. D. Neal, W Wood, and J. Quinn, "Habits—A Repeat Performance," *Current Directions in Psychological Science* 15, no. 4 (2006): 198–202; Judith A. Ouel-lette and Wendy Wood, "Habit and Intention in Everyday Life: The Mul-tiple Processes by Which Past Behavior Predicts Future Behavior," *Psycho-logical Bulletin* 124, no. 1 (1998): 54–74, doi:10.1037//0033-2909.124.1.54; Wendy Wood and David T. Neal, "A New Look at Habits and the Habit-Goal Interface," *Psychological Review* 114, no. 4 (October 2007): 843–63, doi:10.1037/0033-295X.114.4.843.

4. I am oversimplifying a giant research literature on automatic versus con-trolled processing. For an interesting overview, see: J. A. Bargh and M. J.

Ferguson, "Beyond Behaviorism: On the Automaticity of Higher Mental Processes," *Psychological Bulletin* 126, no. 6 (November 2000): 925–45.

5.   Joanna Robertson, "The Pampered Pooches of Paris," BBC, 2011, http://www.bbc.co.uk/news/magazine-16268890.

6.   The dozens of studies showing that our intentions do not predict our behavior very well are documented in a thorough quantitative review: Thomas L. Webb and Paschal Sheeran, "Does Changing Behavioral Intentions Engender Behavior Change? A Meta-Analysis of the Experimental Evidence," *Psychological Bulletin* 132, no. 2 (March 2006): 249–68, doi:10.1037/0033-2909.132.2.249.

7.   Phillippa Lally et al., "How Are Habits Formed: Modelling Habit Formation in the Real World," *European Journal of Social Psychology* 40, no. 6 (October 16, 2010): 998–1009, doi:10.1002/ejsp.674.

8.   Heather Barry Kappes and Gabriele Oettingen, "Positive Fantasies about Idealized Futures Sap Energy," *Journal of Experimental Social Psychology* 47, no. 4 (July 2011): 719–29, doi:10.1016/j.jesp.2011.02.003.

9.   Compared to people who had visualized having already succeeded. Shelley E. Taylor et al., "Harnessing the Imagination: Mental Simulation, Self-Regulation, and Coping," *American Psychologist* 53, no. 4 (1998): 429–39.

10.   Evidence that the performance of one habitual behavior can cue the performance of another: Stef P. J. Kremers, Klazine van der Horst, and Johannes Brug, "Adolescent Screen-Viewing Behaviour Is Associated with Consumption of Sugar-Sweetened Beverages: The Role of Habit Strength and Perceived Parental Norms," *Appetite* 48, no. 3 (May 2007): 345–50, doi:10.1016/j.appet.2006.10.002; Judith A Ouellette and Wendy Wood, "Habit and Intention in Everyday Life: The Multiple Processes by Which Past Behavior Predicts Future Behavior," *Psychological Bulletin* 124, no. 1 (1998): 54–74; Glenn J. Wagner and Gery W. Ryan, "Relationship between Routinization of Daily Behaviors and Medication Adherence in HIV-Positive Drug Users," *AIDS Patient Care and STDs* 18, no. 7 (July 2004): 385–93, doi:10.1089/1087291041518238.

11.   M. Ji and W. Wood, "Purchase and Consumption Habits: Not Necessarily What You Intend," *Journal of Consumer Psychology* 17, no. 4 (October 2007): 261–76, doi:10.1016/S1057-7408(07)70037-2.

12.   This has been shown with exercise, in Wendy Wood, Leona Tam, and Melissa Guerrero Witt, "Changing Circumstances, Disrupting Habits," *Journal of Personality and Social Psychology* 88, no. 6 (2005): 918–33. It's also been shown with making environmentally friendly transportation choices, in Bas Verplanken et al., "Context Change and Travel Mode Choice: Combining the Habit Discontinuity and Self-Activation Hypotheses," *Journal of Environmental Psychology* 28, no. 2 (June 2008): 121–27, doi:10.1016/j.jenvp.2007.10.005. It has not yet been carefully tested with eating, according to Johannes Brug et al., "Environmental Determinants of Healthy Eating: In Need of Theory and Evidence," *Proceedings of the Nutrition Society* 67, no. 3 (August 1, 2008): 307–16, doi:10.1017/S0029665108008616.

13. Jayne Hurley and Bonnie Liebman, "Big: Movie Theaters Fill Buckets . . . and Bellies," *Nutrition Action Health Letter*, December 2009.

14. David T. Neal et al., "The Pull of the Past: When Do Habits Persist Despite Conflict with Motives?," *Personality & Social Psychology Bulletin* 37, no. 11 (November 1, 2011): 1428–37, doi:10.1177/0146167211419863.

15. Don't say I told you to, because movie theaters do not like that.

16. Bas Verplanken and Wendy Wood, "Interventions to Break and Create Consumer Habits," *Journal of Public Policy & Marketing* 25, no. 1 (2006): 90–103.

17. Wood, Tam, and Witt, "Changing Circumstances, Disrupting Habits."

18. Nor do I necessarily recommend eating healthily on vacations. Or perhaps this is a handy rationalization as I happen to be in Paris as I write this and I am eating more than my share of pastries.

19. Peter M. Gollwitzer, "Implementation Intentions: Strong Effects of Simple Plans," *American Psychologist* 54, no. 7 (1999): 493–503.

20. For a review of the evidence, see Peter M. Gollwitzer and Paschal Sheeran, "Implementation Intentions and Goal Achievement: A Meta-Analysis of Effects and Processes" *Advances in Experimental Social Psychology* 38 (2006): 69–119, doi:10.1016/S0065-2601(06)38002-1. A good example can be found in Peter M Gollwitzer and Veronika Brandstätter, "Implementation Intentions and Effective Goal Pursuit," *Journal of Personality and Social Psychology* 73, no. 1 (1997): 186–99.

21. Marieke A. Adriaanse et al., "Do Implementation Intentions Help to Eat a Healthy Diet? A Systematic Review and Meta-Analysis of the Empirical Evidence," *Appetite* 56, no. 1 (February 2011): 183–93, doi:10.1016/j.appet.2010.10.012.

22. Bas Verplanken and Suzanne Faes, "Good Intentions, Bad Habits, and Effects of Forming Implementation Intentions on Healthy Eating," *European Journal of Social Psychology* 29, no. 5–6 (August 1999): 591–604, doi:10.1002/(SICI)1099-0992(199908/09)29:5/6<591::AID-EJSP948>3.0.CO;2-H.

23. Paraphrased from Gollwitzer, "Implementation Intentions." For evidence that implementation intentions help prevent getting derailed by distractions, see Gollwitzer and Sheeran, "Implementation Intentions and Goal Achievement." For evidence that implementation intentions work automatically, see Ute C. Bayer et al., "Responding to Subliminal Cues: Do If-Then Plans Facilitate Action Preparation and Initiation Without Conscious Intent?," *Social Cognition* 27, no. 2 (April 21, 2009): 183–201, doi:10.1521/soco.2009.27.2.183.

24. For evidence that implementation intentions help with the problem of failing to notice or act on an opportunity to fulfill a goal, see Gollwitzer and Sheeran, "Implementation Intentions and Goal Achievement."

25. Janine Chapman, Christopher J. Armitage, and Paul Norman, "Comparing Implementation Intention Interventions in Relation to Young Adults' Intake of Fruit and Vegetables," *Psychology & Health* 24, no. 3 (March 2009): 317–32, doi:10.1080/08870440701864538.

26.   Marieke A. Adriaanse et al., "Planning What Not to Eat: Ironic Effects of Implementation Intentions Negating Unhealthy Habits," *Personality & Social Psychology Bulletin* 37, no. 1 (January 1, 2011): 69–81, doi:10.1177/0146167210390523.

27.   Adriaanse et al., "Do Implementation Intentions Help to Eat a Healthy Diet?"

28.   This study comes from Charlotte Vinkers's dissertation, which I had the pleasure of watching her defend in Utrecht. In Dutch. Charlotte Vinkers, "Future-Oriented Self-Regulation in Eating Behavior" (diss., University of Utrecht, 2013).

29.   This example was mentioned in Molly J. Crockett et al., "Restricting Temptations: Neural Mechanisms of Precommitment," *Neuron* 79, no. 2 (2013): 391–401.

30.   D. Ariely and K. Wertenbroch, "Procrastination, Deadlines, and Performance: Self-Control by Precommitment," *Psychological Science* 13, no. 3 (May 1, 2002): 219–24, doi:10.1111/1467-9280.00441.

31.   Yaacov Trope and Ayelet Fishbach, "Counteractive Self-Control in Overcoming Temptation," *Journal of Personality and Social Psychology* 79, no. 4 (2000): 493–506. Also see the excellently titled article by Xavier Giné, Dean Karlan, and Jonathan Zinman, "Put Your Money Where Your Butt Is: A Commitment Contract for Smoking Cessation," *American Economic Journal: Applied Economics* 2, no. 4 (2010): 213–35.

32.   Janet Schwartz et al., "Healthier by Precommitment," *Psychological Science* 25 (January 3, 2014): 538–46, doi:10.1177/0956797613510950.

33.   George Loewenstein, "Out of Control: Visceral Influences on Behavior," *Organizational Behavior and Human Decision Processes* 65, no. 3 (March 1996): 272–92, doi:10.1006/obhd.1996.0028; Loran F. Nordgren, Frenk van Harreveld, and Joop van der Pligt, "The Restraint Bias: How the Illusion of Self-Restraint Promotes Impulsive Behavior," *Psychological Science* 20, no. 12 (December 1, 2009): 1523–28, doi:10.1111/j.1467-9280.2009.02468.x.

CHAPTER 10: HOW TO COMFORT AN ASTRONAUT

1.   NASA publishes its evidence in Michele Perchonok and Grace Douglas, "Risk Factor of Inadequate Food System," in *Human Health Performance Risks of Space Exploration Missions: Evidence Reviewed by the NASA Human Research Program*, ed. Jancy C. McPhee and John B. Charles (Houston: NASA, 2009), 295–316.

2.   Charles T. Bourland and Gregory L. Vogt, *The Astronaut's Cookbook: Tales, Recipes, and More* (New York: Springer International, 2009).

3.   B. J. Caldwell et al., "Fluid Shift to the Upper Body Reduces Nasal Cavity Dimension and Airflow in Head-Down Bed Rest Subjects," in *NASA Human Research Program Investigators' Workshop* (Houston, 2012).

4.   Barb Stuckey, *Taste: Surprising Stories and Science About why Food Tastes Good* (New York: Simon & Schuster, 2012).

5. Perchonok and Douglas, "Risk Factor of Inadequate Food System."

6. See, for example: D. J. Wallis and M. M. Hetherington, "Emotions and Eating. Self-Reported and Experimentally Induced Changes in Food Intake under Stress," *Appetite* 52, no. 2 (April 2009): 355–62, doi:10.1016/j .appet.2008.11.007. For a review, see: C. Greeno and R Wing, "Stress-Induced Eating," *Psychological Bulletin* 115 (1994): 444.

7. J. McPhee and J. Charles, eds., *Human Health Performance Risks of Space Exploration Missions: Evidence Reviewed by the NASA Human Research Program* (Houston: NASA, 2009).

8. Joe Redden and Zata Vickers, along with our graduate students Heather Wagner, Rachel Burns, and Katie Osdoba, and lab manager Britt Ahlstrom.

9. Well, nobody had ever tested it the way we thought it should be done—by giving people their own idiosyncratic comfort food, though there is one rigorous test of chocolate on moods: Michael Macht and Jochen Mueller, "Immediate Effects of Chocolate on Experimentally Induced Mood States," *Appetite* 49, no. 3 (November 2007): 667–74, doi:10.1016/j.appet.2007.05.004.

10. This shows just how strongly we believed in the ability of comfort food to improve mood.

11. Britt Ahlstrom, my lab manager at the time, deserves all the credit for finding the foods.

12. The four comfort food studies described in this chapter are published in Heather Wagner et al., "The Myth of Comfort Food," *Health Psychology* (2014).

13. The research methodologists among you might be wondering if we had simply improved their moods as far as it was possible to improve them, leaving no "room" for comfort food to outperform the other food, called a ceiling effect. This was not the case, as we show most clearly in the fourth study in the article.

14. There may be chemical properties of chocolate that cause it to make you feel good over a longer amount of time, but not immediately, the way we all expect comfort food to work. For a review, see Andrew Scholey and Lauren Owen, "Effects of Chocolate on Cognitive Function and Mood: A Systematic Review," *Nutrition Reviews* 71, no. 10 (October 2013): 665–81, doi:10.1111/ nure.12065.

15. Wagner et al., "The Myth of Comfort Food."

16. This is a popular comfort food among astronauts.

17. There are people who are particularly likely to seek out comfort food or to eat when they feel bad. They are called emotional eaters. There is no evidence that comfort food helps them more than it does any other eaters. A measure of this appears in Tatjana van Strien et al., "The Dutch Eating Behavior Questionnaire (DEBQ) for Assessment of Restrained, Emotional, and External Eating Behavior," *International Journal of Eating Disorders* 5, no. 2 (February 1986): 295–315, doi:10.1002/1098-108X(198602)5:2<295::AID-EAT2260050209>3.0.CO;2-T.

18. Meryl P. Gardner et al., "Better Moods for Better Eating? How Mood Influences Food Choice," *Journal of Consumer Psychology* (January 2014),

doi:10.1016/j.jcps.2014.01.002.

19.   Yann Cornil and Pierre Chandon, "From Fan to Fat? Vicarious Los-
       ing Increases Unhealthy Eating, but Self-Affirmation Is an Effective
       Remedy," *Psychological Science* 24, no. 10 (October 1, 2013): 1936–46,
       doi:10.1177/0956797613481232.

20.   Michael Macht, Jessica Meininger, and Jochen Roth, "The Pleasures of
       Eating: A Qualitative Analysis," *Journal of Happiness Studies* 6, no. 2 (June
       2005): 137–60, doi:10.1007/s10902-005-0287-x; Jordi Quoidbach et al.,
       "Positive Emotion Regulation and Well-Being: Comparing the Impact of
       Eight Savoring and Dampening Strategies," *Personality and Individual Dif-
       ferences* 49, no. 5 (October 2010): 368–73, doi:10.1016/j.paid.2010.03.048.

21.   E. K. Papies, L. W. Barsalou, and R. Custers, "Mindful Attention Prevents
       Mindless Impulses," *Social Psychological and Personality Science* 3, no. 3 (Au-
       gust 29, 2011): 291–99, doi:10.1177/1948550611419031. Also see P. Rozin
       et al., "The Ecology of Eating: Smaller Portion Sizes in France Than in the
       United States Help Explain the French Paradox," *Psychological Science* 14, no.
       5 (September 1, 2003): 450–54, doi:10.1111/1467-9280.02452.

22.   This is true for dieters or people trying not to eat, as Andrew Ward and I
       found in our early eating studies. Ward and Mann, "Don't Mind If I Do:
       Disinhibited Eating Under Cognitive Load," April 1, 2000; Traci Mann and
       Andrew Ward, "To Eat or Not to Eat: Implications of the Attentional Myo-
       pia Model for Restrained Eaters," *Journal of Abnormal Psychology* 113, no. 1
       (2004): 90–98.

23.   Reine C. van der Wal and Lotte F. van Dillen, "Leaving a Flat Taste in Your
       Mouth: Task Load Reduces Taste Perception," *Psychological Science* 24, no. 7
       (July 1, 2013): 1277–84, doi:10.1177/0956797612471953.

24.   There is a slight difference. Intuitive eaters specifically reject following diet
       rules or plans and only eat what their body "tells" them it wants. Mindful
       eaters might follow an eating plan, so long as they are attentive to their eating
       and hunger. For specific measures of each, see Tracy L. Tylka, "Develop-
       ment and Psychometric Evaluation of a Measure of Intuitive Eating," *Journal
       of Counseling Psychology* 53, no. 2 (2006): 226–40; Celia Framson et al.,
       "Development and Validation of the Mindful Eating Questionnaire," *Jour-
       nal of the American Dietetic Association* 109, no. 8 (August 2009): 1439–44,
       doi:10.1016/j.jada.2009.05.006.

25.   For an example, see Gayle M. Timmerman and Adama Brown, "The Ef-
       fect of a Mindful Restaurant Eating Intervention on Weight Management
       in Women," *Journal of Nutrition Education and Behavior* 44, no. 1 (Janu-
       ary 2012): 22–28, doi:10.1016/j.jneb.2011.03.143. For a review, see G. A.
       O'Reilly et al., "Mindfulness-Based Interventions for Obesity-Related Eat-
       ing Behaviours: A Literature Review," *Obesity Reviews* (March 18, 2014),
       doi:10.1111/obr.12156.

26.   Linda Bacon et al., "Size Acceptance and Intuitive Eating Improve Health for
       Obese, Female Chronic Dieters," *Journal of the American Dietetic Association*
       105, no. 6 (June 2005): 929–36, doi:10.1016/j.jada.2005.03.011.

27.   This was found in two of the three studies reviewed in O'Reilly et al., "Mindfulness-Based Interventions for Obesity-Related Eating Behaviours."

28.   Megan Spanjers, "A Nutritious Diet Without Calorie Counting and Restrictive Rules? An Analysis of Nutrition Trends among Intuitive Eaters," (University of Minnesota, 2013).

29.   This is shown in 11 out of 12 studies in O'Reilly et al., "Mindfulness-Based Interventions for Obesity-Related Eating Behaviours." For an example, see Jean Kristeller, Ruth Q. Wolever, and Virgil Sheets, "Mindfulness-Based Eating Awareness Training (MB-EAT) for Binge Eating: A Randomized Clinical Trial," *Mindfulness* (February 1, 2013), doi:10.1007/s12671-012-0179-1.

30.   P. Rozin et al., "Attitudes to Food and the Role of Food in Life in the U.S.A., Japan, Flemish Belgium and France: Possible Implications for the Diet-Health Debate," *Appetite* 33, no. 2 (October 1999): 163–80, doi:10.1006/appe.1999.0244.

31.   My kids call this behavior "the commercial chew."

32.   Rozin et al., "The Ecology of Eating."

33.   Rozin et al., "Attitudes to Food and the Role of Food in Life in the U.S.A., Japan, Flemish Belgium and France."

34.   Ibid.

35.   Jordi Quoidbach et al., "Money Giveth, Money Taketh Away: The Dual Effect of Wealth on Happiness," *Psychological Science* 21, no. 6 (June 1, 2010): 759–63, doi:10.1177/0956797610371963.

36.   Ibid.

37.   Richard Kirshenbaum, "Let Them Eat Kale: Extreme Dieters Ruining Dinner Parties for Everyone Else. Two Almonds Is Now Considered a Meal?," *New York Observer*, January 21, 2014.

CHAPTER 11: WHY TO STOP OBSESSING AND BE OKAY WITH YOUR BODY

1.   Art Caplan, "New Zealand's Solution for Rising Health Costs? Deport Fat People," NBC News, 2013, http://www.nbcnews.com/health/diet-fitness/new-zealands-solution-rising-health-costs-deport-fat-people-f6C10861122.

2.   Helen Carter, "Too Fat to Adopt—the Married, Teetotal Couple Rejected by Council Because of Man's Weight," *Guardian*, January 16, 2009.

3.   Mark V. Roehling et al., "The Effects of Weight Bias on Job-Related Outcomes: A Meta-Analysis of Experimental Studies," in Academy of Management Annual Meeting, Anaheim, CA, 2008.

4.   M. V. Roehling, P. V. Roehling, and L. M. Odland, "Investigating the Validity of Stereotypes about Overweight Employees: The Relationship between Body Weight and Normal Personality Traits," *Group & Organization Management* 33, no. 4 (May 28, 2008): 392–424, doi:10.1177/1059601108321518.

5.   Brian A. Nosek et al., "Pervasiveness and Correlates of Implicit Attitudes and Stereotypes," *European Review of Social Psychology* 18, no. 1 (January 2007):

36–88, doi:10.1080/10463280701489053. Sixty-nine percent of participants implicitly preferred thin people over obese people.

6.   Ibid.

7.   R. T. Azevedo et al., "Weighing the Stigma of Weight: An fMRI Study of Neural Reactivity to the Pain of Obese Individuals," *NeuroImage* 91 (May 1, 2014): 109–19, doi:10.1016/j.neuroimage.2013.11.041. ⸱

8.   R. M. Puhl, T. Andreyeva, and K. D. Brownell, "Perceptions of Weight Discrimination: Prevalence and Comparison to Race and Gender Discrimination in America," *International Journal of Obesity* 32, no. 6 (2008): 992–1000, doi:10.1038/ijo.2008.22.

9.   Puhl and Heuer, "The Stigma of Obesity: A Review and Update," 2009.

10. Examples of the above, for college admissions, see Jane Wardle, Jo Waller, and Martin J. Jarvis, "Sex Differences in the Association of Socioeconomic Status with Obesity," *American Journal of Public Health* 92, no. 8 (August 10, 2002): 1299–1304, doi:10.2105/AJPH.92.8.1299. For health insurance, see Walter Hamilton, "Report: CVS Caremark Demands Workers Disclose Weight, Health Info," *Los Angeles Times*, March 20, 2013.

11. Legal remedies are reviewed, and new laws suggested, in Young Suh et al., "Support for Laws to Prohibit Weight Discrimination in the United States: Public Attitudes from 2011 to 2013," *Obesity* (Silver Spring, MD) 22, no.8 (April 8, 2014):1872–9, doi:10.1002/oby.20750.

12. For boys, see Nina Karnehed et al., "Obesity and Attained Education: Cohort Study of More than 700,000 Swedish Men," *Obesity* (Silver Spring, MD) 14, no. 8 (August 2006): 1421–28, doi:10.1038/oby.2006.161. For girls but not boys: R. Crosnoe, "Gender, Obesity, and Education," *Sociology of Education* 80, no. 3 (July 1, 2007): 241–60, doi:10.1177/003804070708000303. For girls and boys, but these researchers did not control for intelligence: Wardle, Waller, and Jarvis, "Sex Differences in the Association of Socioeconomic Status with Obesity."

13. Jacob M Burmeister et al., "Weight Bias in Graduate School Admissions," *Obesity* (Silver Spring, MD) 21, no. 5 (May 2013): 918–20, doi:10.1002/oby.20171.

14. For a review, see R. Puhl and C. Heuer, "The Stigma of Obesity: A Review and Update," *Obesity* 17, no. 5 (2009): 941–64.

15. Scott Klarenbach et al., "Population-Based Analysis of Obesity and Workforce Participation," *Obesity* (Silver Spring, MD) 14, no. 5 (May 2006): 920–27, doi:10.1038/oby.2006.106.

16. Roehling et al., "The Effects of Weight Bias on Job-Related Outcomes."

17. K. S. O'Brien et al., "Obesity Discrimination: The Role of Physical Appearance, Personal Ideology, and Anti-Fat Prejudice," *International Journal of Obesity* 37, no. 3 (March 2013): 455–60, doi:10.1038/ijo.2012.52.

18. Klarenbach et al., "Population-Based Analysis of Obesity and Workforce Participation."

19. They rescinded the policy after getting unfavorable media attention. James Zervios, "Texas-Based Hospital 'Citizens Medical Center' Suspends Body

Mass Index Employment Requirement," *Obesity Action Coalition*, 2012, http://www.obesityaction.org/newsroom/news-releases/2012-news-releases/texas-based-hospital-citizens-medical-center-suspends-body-mass-index-employment-requirement.

20.   Roehling et al., "The Effects of Weight Bias on Job-Related Outcomes."

21.   For a thorough discussion, see Chapter 6 of Terry Poulton, *No Fat Chicks*: *How Big Business Profits by Making Women Hate Their Bodies—And How to Fight Back* (New York: Birch Lane Press, 1997).

22.   Ibid.

23.   Charles L. Baum and William F. Ford, "The Wage Effects of Obesity: A Longitudinal Study," *Health Economics* 13, no. 9 (September 2004): 885–99, doi:10.1002/hec.881. For similar data from Europe, see Giorgio Brunello and Béatrice D'Hombres, "Does Body Weight Affect Wages? Evidence from Europe," *Economics and Human Biology* 5, no. 1 (March 2007): 1–19, doi:10.1016/j.ehb.2006.11.002.

24.   Timothy A. Judge and Daniel M. Cable, "When It Comes to Pay, Do the Thin Win? The Effect of Weight on Pay for Men and Women," *Journal of Applied Psychology* 96, no. 1 (January 1, 2011): 95–112, doi:10.1037/a0020860.

25.   Baum and Ford, "The Wage Effects of Obesity."

26.   Patricia V. Roehling et al., "Weight Discrimination and the Glass Ceiling Effect among Top US CEOs," *Equal Opportunities International* 28, no. 2 (February 13, 2009): 179–96, doi:10.1108/02610150910937916.

27.   Patricia V. Roehling et al., "Weight Bias in US Candidate Selection and Election," *Equality, Diversity and Inclusion* 33, no. 4 (May 13, 2014): 334–46, doi:10.1108/EDI-10-2013-0081.

28.   N. A. Schvey et al., "The Influence of a Defendant's Body Weight on Perceptions of Guilt," *International Journal of Obesity (2005)* 37, no. 9 (September 2013): 1275–81, doi:10.1038/ijo.2012.211.

29.   Jason D. Seacat, Sarah C. Dougal, and Dooti Roy, "A Daily Diary Assessment of Female Weight Stigmatization," *Journal of Health Psychology* (March 18, 2014): 1359105314525067–, doi:10.1177/1359105314525067.

30.   See also Puhl and Brownell, "Confronting and Coping with Weight Stigma."

31.   Michael Scherer, "The Elephant in the Room: How Chris Christie Can Win Over the GOP," *Time*, November 18, 2013.

32.   Puhl and Brownell, "Confronting and Coping with Weight Stigma."

33.   See Chapter 4 of Poulton, *No Fat Chicks*. Also see Lesley, "What's Wrong with Fat-Shaming?," XOJane.com, 2012, http://www.xojane.com/issues/whats-wrong-fat-shaming. This beautifully written and heartbreaking column is worth reading in full.

34.   Poulton, *No Fat Chicks*; Lesley, "What's Wrong With Fat-Shaming?"

35.   For example, see Rod Liddle, "If We Don't Stigmatise Fat People, There'll Be Lots More of Them," *Spectator*, October 19, 2013.

36.   Daniel Callahan, "Obesity: Chasing an Elusive Epidemic," *Hastings Center Report* 43, no. 1 (2013): 34–40, doi:10.1002/hast.114. He also argues that stigmatizing smokers was partly responsible for reductions in smoking in the

last few decades. It's not clear if that is true, but even if it is, that doesn't mean it would work for obesity (and the evidence in this part of the chapter shows it does not).

37. Liddle, "If We Don't Stigmatise Fat People, There'll Be Lots More of Them."

38. Brenda Major et al., "The Ironic Effects of Weight Stigma," *Journal of Experimental Social Psychology* 51 (March 2014): 74–80, doi:10.1016/j .jesp.2013.11.009.

39. Other studies show this as well. See Elizabeth A. Pascoe and Laura Smart Richman, "Effect of Discrimination on Food Decisions," *Self and Identity* 10, no. 3 (July 2011): 396–406, doi:10.1080/15298868.2010.526384; Natasha A. Schvey, Rebecca M. Puhl, and Kelly D. Brownell, "The Impact of Weight Stigma on Caloric Consumption," *Obesity* (Silver Spring, MD) 19, no. 10 (October 2011): 1957–62, doi:10.1038/oby.2011.204; Rebecca Puhl, Joerg Luedicke, and Jamie Lee Peterson, "Public Reactions to Obesity-Related Health Campaigns: A Randomized Controlled Trial," *American Journal of Preventive Medicine* 45, no. 1 (July 1, 2013): 36–48, doi:10.1016/ j.amepre.2013.02.010.

40. Lenny R. Vartanian and Sarah A. Novak, "Internalized Societal Attitudes Moderate the Impact of Weight Stigma on Avoidance of Exercise," *Obesity* (Silver Spring, MD) 19, no. 4 (April 2011): 757–62, doi:10.1038/ oby.2010.234; Lenny R. Vartanian and Jacqueline G. Shaprow, "Effects of Weight Stigma on Exercise Motivation and Behavior: A Preliminary Investigation among College-Aged Females," *Journal of Health Psychology* 13, no. 1 (January 1, 2008): 131–38, doi:10.1177/1359105307084318.

41. Jason D. Seacat and Kristin D. Mickelson, "Stereotype Threat and the Exercise/Dietary Health Intentions of Overweight Women," *Journal of Health Psychology* 14, no. 4 (May 1, 2009): 556–67, doi:10.1177/1359105309103575.

42. Vartanian and Shaprow, "Effects of Weight Stigma on Exercise Motivation and Behavior"; Vartanian and Novak, "Internalized Societal Attitudes Moderate the Impact of Weight Stigma on Avoidance of Exercise."

43. Technically, it prevented an expected decrease in cortisol: Schvey, Puhl, and Brownell, "The Stress of Stigma." Also see Tomiyama et al., "Associations of Weight Stigma with Cortisol and Oxidative Stress Independent of Adiposity."

44. Only 5 percent of lead characters on television shows are played by obese people, and in movies, obese actors and actresses aren't even necessarily hired to play obese characters. Bradley S. Greenberg et al., "Portrayals of Overweight and Obese Individuals on Commercial Television," *American Journal of Public Health* 93, no. 8 (August 10, 2003): 1342–48, doi:10.2105/ AJPH.93.8.1342.

45. Jeffrey M. Hunger and A. Janet Tomiyama, "Weight Labeling and Obesity," *JAMA Pediatrics* (April 28, 2014), doi:10.1001/jamapediatrics.2014.122. For similar findings with adults, see Angelina R. Sutin and Antonio Terracciano, "Perceived Weight Discrimination and Obesity," ed. Robert L. Newton, *PloS One* 8, no. 7 (January 2013): e70048, doi:10.1371/journal.pone.0070048.

46.   Flegal et al., "Prevalence of Obesity and Trends in the Distribution of Body Mass Index among US Adults, 1999–2010."

47.   Tatiana Andreyeva, Rebecca M. Puhl, and Kelly D. Brownell, "Changes in Perceived Weight Discrimination among Americans, 1995–1996 through 2004–2006," *Obesity* (Silver Spring, MD) 16, no. 5 (May 2008): 1129–34, doi:10.1038/oby.2008.35.

48.   Gordon W. Allport, *The Nature of Prejudice* (Reading, MA: Addison-Wesley, 1954). For the specific example of homophobia, see Sebastian E. Barto, Israel Berger, and Peter Hegarty, "Interventions to Reduce Sexual Prejudice: A Study-Space Analysis and Meta-Analytic Review," *Journal of Sex Research* 51, no. 4 (January 2014): 363–82, doi:10.1080/00224499.2013.871625.

49.   S. S. Wang, K. D. Brownell, and T. A. Wadden, "The Influence of the Stigma of Obesity on Overweight Individuals," *International Journal of Obesity and Related Metabolic Disorders* 28, no. 10 (October 1, 2004): 1333–7, doi:10.1038/sj.ijo.0802730.

50.   Tracy Moore, "I Don't Love (or Hate) My Body—and So Can You!," Jezebel.com, 2014, http://jezebel.com/i-dont-love-or-hate-my-body-and-so-can-you-1557099034.

51.   Joan Jacobs Brumberg, *The Body Project*: *An Intimate History of American Girls* (New York: Vintage Books, 1998).

52.   Ibid.

53.   "Gym, Health & Fitness Clubs in the US: Market Research Report," IBISWorld.com, 2014, http://www.ibisworld.com/industry/default.aspx?indid=1655.

54.   Se-Jin Lee, "Regulation of Muscle Mass by Myostatin," *Annual Review of Cell and Developmental Biology* 20 (January 8, 2004): 61–86, doi:10.1146/annurev.cellbio.20.012103.135836.

55.   Frank Bruni, "These Wretched Vessels," *New York Times*, December 24, 2012.

CHAPTER 12: THE REAL REASONS TO EXERCISE AND STRATEGIES FOR STICKING WITH IT

1.   A strong case is made by Amy Luke and Richard S Cooper, "Physical Activity Does Not Influence Obesity Risk: Time to Clarify the Public Health Message," *International Journal of Epidemiology* 42, no. 6 (December 1, 2013): 1831–36, doi:10.1093/ije/dyt159. Also see the following for a rebuttal: James O Hill and John C. Peters, "Commentary: Physical Activity and Weight Control," *International Journal of Epidemiology* 42, no. 6 (December 1, 2013): 1840–42, doi:10.1093/ije/dyt161.

2.   This point is presented as one of nine facts about obesity in Casazza et al., "Myths, Presumptions, and Facts about Obesity."

3.   Petra Stiegler and Adam Cunliffe, "The Role of Diet and Exercise for the Maintenance of Fat-Free Mass and Resting Metabolic Rate during Weight Loss," *Sports Medicine* (Auckland, NZ) 36, no. 3 (January 2006): 239–62.

4.   N. A. King et al., "The Interaction between Exercise, Appetite, and Food
     Intake: Implications for Weight Control," *American Journal of Lifestyle Med-
     icine* 7, no. 4 (February 6, 2013): 265–73, doi:10.1177/1559827613475584;
     Catia Martins et al., "Effects of Exercise on Gut Peptides, Energy Intake
     and Appetite," *Journal of Endocrinology* 193, no. 2 (May 1, 2007): 251–58,
     doi:10.1677/JOE-06-0030.

5.   Carolina O. C. Werle, Brian Wansink, and Collin R. Payne, "Just Think-
     ing about Exercise Makes Me Serve More Food: Physical Activity and Cal-
     orie Compensation," *Appetite* 56, no. 2 (April 2011): 332–35, doi:10.1016/j
     .appet.2010.12.016.

6.   The government recommends 150 minutes of moderate exercise (or 75 of in-
     tense exercise) per week for health, but 300 minutes of moderate exercise per
     week (or 150 minutes of intense exercise) for weight loss. U.S. Department of
     Health and Human Services, "2008 Physical Activity Guidelines for Ameri-
     cans," http://www.health.gov/paguidelines/.

7.   This comes from a review of eighty studies that included over a million par-
     ticipants. About half of the studies made a point of controlling for weight.
     Guenther Samitz, Matthias Egger, and Marcel Zwahlen, "Domains of Physi-
     cal Activity and All-Cause Mortality: Systematic Review and Dose-Response
     Meta-Analysis of Cohort Studies," *International Journal of Epidemiology* 40,
     no. 5 (October 1, 2011): 1382–400, doi:10.1093/ije/dyr112.

8.   These patients were followed for over eight years. Edward W Gregg et al.,
     "Relationship of Walking to Mortality among US Adults with Diabetes," *Ar-
     chives of Internal Medicine* 163, no. 12 (June 23, 2003): 1440–7, doi:10.1001/
     archinte.163.12.1440.

9.   Samitz, Egger, and Zwahlen, "Domains of Physical Activity and All-Cause
     Mortality."

10. Huseyin Naci and John P. A. Ioannidis, "Comparative Effectiveness of Ex-
     ercise and Drug Interventions on Mortality Outcomes: Metaepidemiological
     Study," *BMJ* (Clinical Research Ed.) 347 (January 2013): f5577.

11. Ibid.

12. Mark Hamer, Kim L. Lavoie, and Simon L. Bacon, "Taking Up Physical
     Activity in Later Life and Healthy Ageing: The English Longitudinal Study
     of Ageing," *British Journal of Sports Medicine* 48, no. 3 (February 1, 2014):
     239–43, doi:10.1136/bjsports-2013-092993.

13. Francesco Sofi et al., "Physical Activity during Leisure Time and Primary
     Prevention of Coronary Heart Disease: An Updated Meta-Analysis of Co-
     hort Studies," *European Journal of Cardiovascular Prevention and Rehabilita-
     tion* 15, no. 3 (June 1, 2008): 247–57, doi:10.1097/HJR.0b013e3282f232ac.

14. Chong Do Lee, Aaron R. Folsom, and Steven N. Blair, "Physical Activity
     and Stroke Risk: A Meta-Analysis," *Stroke* 34, no. 10 (October 1, 2003):
     2475–81, doi:10.1161/01.STR.0000091843.02517.9D.

15. Frank B. Hu et al., "Walking Compared with Vigorous Physical Activity
     and Risk of Type 2 Diabetes in Women," *JAMA* 282, no. 15 (October 20,
     1999): 1433, doi:10.1001/jama.282.15.1433; S. P. Helmrich et al., "Physical

Activity and Reduced Occurrence of Non-Insulin-Dependent Diabetes Mellitus," *New England Journal of Medicine* 325, no. 3 (July 18, 1991): 147–52, doi:10.1056/NEJM199107183250302; Bridget M. Kuehn, "Physical Activity May Stave Off Diabetes for Women at Risk," *JAMA{dec63}* 311, no. 22 (June 11, 2014): 2263, doi:10.1001/jama.2014.6862.

16.   Inger Thune and Anne-Sofie Furberg, "Physical Activity and Cancer Risk: Dose-Response and Cancer, All Sites and Site-Specific," *Medicine and Science in Sports and Exercise* 33, Suppl. (June 1, 2001): S530–S550, doi:10.1097/00005768-200106001-00025.

17.   This was true regardless of whether they lost weight. Sean Carroll and Mike Dudfield, "What Is the Relationship between Exercise and Metabolic Abnormalities?," *Sports Medicine* 34, no. 6 (2004): 371–418, doi:10.2165/00007256-200434060-00004.

18.   Kelly M. Naugle, Roger B. Fillingim, and Joseph L. Riley, "A Meta-Analytic Review of the Hypoalgesic Effects of Exercise," *Journal of Pain* 13, no. 12 (December 2012): 1139–50, doi:10.1016/j.jpain.2012.09.006.

19.   Liisa Byberg et al., "Total Mortality After Changes in Leisure Time Physical Activity in 50 Year Old Men: 35 Year Follow-up of Population Based Cohort," *BMJ* (Clinical Research Ed.) 338, no. mar05_2 (January 5, 2009): b688, doi:10.1136/bmj.b688.

20.   Caudwell et al., "Exercise Alone Is Not Enough."

21.   Ibid.

22.   This is presented as one of nine facts about obesity in Casazza et al., "Myths, Presumptions, and Facts about Obesity."

23.   Petri Wiklund et al., "Metabolic Response to 6-Week Aerobic Exercise Training and Dieting in Previously Sedentary Overweight and Obese Pre-Menopausal Women: A Randomized Trial," *Journal of Sport and Health Science* (June 2014), doi:10.1016/j.jshs.2014.03.013.

24.   Organisation for Economic Co-operation and Development Better Life Index, 2014, Center for Economic and Policy Research, http://www.cepr.net/index.php/publications/reports/no-vacation-nation-2013.

25.   Rebecca Ray, Milla Sanes, and John Schmitt, *No-Vacation Nation Revisited* (Washington, DC: Center for Economic and Policy Research, 2013).

26.   The overall evidence for the effects of stress on health is summarized in the thorough and readable book by Robert Sapolsky, *Why Zebras Don't Get Ulcers*, 3rd ed. (New York: Holt Paperbacks, 2004). The classic scholarly review is McEwen and Seeman, "Protective and Damaging Effects of Mediators of Stress."

27.   This is nicely demonstrated in studies of parachute jumps, for example, Manfred Schedlowski et al., "Changes of Natural Killer Cells during Acute Psychological Stress," *Journal of Clinical Immunology* 13, no. 2 (March 1993): 119–26, doi:10.1007/BF00919268.

28.   S. Cohen, D. Janicki-Deverts, and G. E. Miller, "Psychological Stress and Disease," *JAMA* 298, no. 14 (2007): 1685–87, doi:10.1001/jama.298.14.1685.

29.   Sapolsky, *Why Zebras Don't Get Ulcers*.

30.   Ibid.

31. Ibid.

32. Sally S. Dickerson and Margaret E. Kemeny, "Acute Stressors and Cortisol Responses: A Theoretical Integration and Synthesis of Laboratory Research," *Psychological Bulletin* 130, no. 3 (May 1, 2004): 355–91, doi:10.1037/003 3-2909.130.3.355; Gregory E. Miller, Edith Chen, and Eric S. Zhou, "If It Goes Up, Must It Come Down? Chronic Stress and the Hypothalamic-Pituitary-Adrenocortical Axis in Humans," *Psychological Bulletin* 133, no. 1 (2007): 25–45.

33. P. Bjorntorp, "Do Stress Reactions Cause Abdominal Obesity and Comorbidities?," *Obesity Reviews* 2, no. 2 (May 2001): 73–86, doi:10.1046/j.1467 789x.2001.00027.x; E. S Epel et al., "Stress and Body Shape: Stress-Induced Cortisol Secretion Is Consistently Greater among Women with Central Fat," *Psychosomatic Medicine* 62, no. 5 (2000): 623–32.

34. Suzanne C. Segerstrom and Gregory E. Miller, "Psychological Stress and the Human Immune System: A Meta-Analytic Study of 30 Years of Inquiry," *Psychological Bulletin* 130, no. 4 (July 1, 2004): 601–30, doi:10.1037 /0033-2909.130.4.601; Theodore F. Robles, Ronald Glaser, and Janice K. Kiecolt-Glaser, "Out of Balance. A New Look at Chronic Stress, Depression, and Immunity," *Current Directions in Psychological Science* 14, no. 2 (April 2005): 111–15, doi:10.1111/j.0963-7214.2005.00345.x; Schedlowski et al., "Changes of Natural Killer Cells during Acute Psychological Stress."

35. Sheldon Cohen, David A. Tyrrell, and Andrew P. Smith, "Psychological Stress and Susceptibility to the Common Cold," *New England Journal of Medicine* 325, no. 9 (1991): 606–12.

36. Jessica Walburn et al., "Psychological Stress and Wound Healing in Humans: A Systematic Review and Meta-Analysis," *Journal of Psychosomatic Research* 67, no. 3 (September 2009): 253–71, doi:10.1016/j.jpsychores.2009.04.002.

37. Elissa S. Epel et al., "Accelerated Telomere Shortening in Response to Life Stress," *Proceedings of the National Academy of Sciences of the United States of America* 101, no. 49 (December 7, 2004): 17312–15, doi:10.1073/ pnas.0407162101.

38. Kimberly A. Brownley et al., "Sympathoadrenergic Mechanisms in Reduced Hemodynamic Stress Responses After Exercise," *Medicine and Science in Sports and Exercise* 35, no. 6 (June 2003): 978–86, doi:10.1249/01. MSS.0000069335.12756.1B.

39. Peter Salmon, "Effects of Physical Exercise on Anxiety, Depression, and Sensitivity to Stress," *Clinical Psychology Review* 21, no. 1 (February 2001): 33–61, doi:10.1016/S0272-7358(99)00032-X.

40. Cheryl J. Hansen, Larry C. Stevens, and J. Richard Coast, "Exercise Duration and Mood State: How Much Is Enough to Feel Better?," *Health Psychology* 20, no. 4 (July 1, 2001): 267–75, doi:10.1037/0278-6133.20.4.267.

41. J. C. Coulson, J. McKenna, and M. Field, "Exercising at Work and Self-Reported Work Performance," *International Journal of Workplace Health Management* 1, no. 3 (September 26, 2008): 176–97, doi:10.1108/17538350810926534; Robert R. Yeung, "The Acute Effects of

Exercise on Mood State," *Journal of Psychosomatic Research* 40, no. 2 (February 1996): 123–41, doi:10.1016/0022-3999(95)00554-4.

42.   Salmon, "Effects of Physical Exercise on Anxiety, Depression, and Sensitivity to Stress."

43.   Steven J. Petruzzello et al., "A Meta-Analysis on the Anxiety-Reducing Effects of Acute and Chronic Exercise," *Sports Medicine* 11, no. 3 (March 1991): 143–82, doi:10.2165/00007256-199111030-00002.

44.   Peter J. Carek, Sarah E. Laibstain, and Stephen M. Carek, "Exercise for the Treatment of Depression and Anxiety," *International Journal of Psychiatry in Medicine* 41, no. 1 (January 1, 2011): 15–28, doi:10.2190/PM.41.1.c; Andreas Broocks et al., "Comparison of Aerobic Exercise, Clomipramine, and Placebo in the Treatment of Panic Disorder," *American Journal of Psychiatry* 155, no. 5 (May 1, 1998): 603–9.

45.   Carek, Laibstain, and Carek, "Exercise for the Treatment of Depression and Anxiety"; Gillian E. Mead et al., "Exercise for Depression," *Cochrane Database of Systematic Reviews* no. 4 (January 2008): CD004366, doi:10.1002/14651858.CD004366.pub3.

46.   Hamer, Lavoie, and Bacon, "Taking Up Physical Activity in Later Life and Healthy Ageing."

47.   Daniel Y. T. Fong et al., "Physical Activity for Cancer Survivors: Meta-Analysis of Randomised Controlled Trials," *BMJ* (Clinical Research Ed.) 344, no. jan30_5 (January 31, 2012): e70, doi:10.1136/bmj.e70.

48.   M E. Hopkins et al., "Differential Effects of Acute and Regular Physical Exercise on Cognition and Affect," *Neuroscience* 215 (July 26, 2012): 59–68, doi:10.1016/j.neuroscience.2012.04.056; Hamer, Lavoie, and Bacon, "Taking Up Physical Activity in Later Life and Healthy Ageing"; Maria A. I. Aberg et al., "Cardiovascular Fitness Is Associated with Cognition in Young Adulthood," *Proceedings of the National Academy of Sciences of the United States of America* 106, no. 49 (December 8, 2009): 20906–11, doi:10.1073/pnas.0905307106; Arthur F. Kramer, Kirk I. Erickson, and Stanley J. Colcombe, "Exercise, Cognition, and the Aging Brain," *Journal of Applied Physiology* 101, no. 4 (October 1, 2006): 1237–42, doi:10.1152/japplphysiol.00500.2006.

49.   Kate Lambourne and Phillip Tomporowski, "The Effect of Exercise-Induced Arousal on Cognitive Task Performance: A Meta-Regression Analysis," *Brain Research* 1341 (June 23, 2010): 12–24, doi:10.1016/j.brainres.2010.03.091.

50.   Marily Oppezzo and Daniel L. Schwartz, "Give Your Ideas Some Legs: The Positive Effect of Walking on Creative Thinking," *Journal of Experimental Psychology* (2014).

51.   Shelley S. Tworoger et al., "Effects of a Yearlong Moderate-Intensity Exercise and a Stretching Intervention on Sleep Quality in Postmenopausal Women," *Sleep* 26, no. 7 (2003): 830–38.

52.   Abby C. King et al., "Moderate-Intensity Exercise and Self-Rated Quality of Sleep in Older Adults," *JAMA* 277, no. 1 (January 1, 1997): 32–37, doi:10.1001/jama.1997.03540250040029.

53. This study did not control for weight or weight loss. Hamer, Lavoie, and Bacon, "Taking Up Physical Activity in Later Life and Healthy Ageing."

54. B. L. Tracy et al., "Muscle Quality. II. Effects of Strength Training in 65- to 75-Yr-Old Men and Women," *Journal of Applied Physiology* 86, no. 1 (January 1, 1999): 195–201.

55. Kramer, Erickson, and Colcombe, "Exercise, Cognition, and the Aging Brain."

56. U.S. Department of Health and Human Services, "2008 Physical Activity Guidelines for Americans."

57. Your maximum heart rate can be calculated here: http://www.ntnu.edu/cerg/hrmax.

58. Karissa L. Canning et al., "Individuals Underestimate Moderate and Vigorous Intensity Physical Activity," ed. Conrad P. Earnest, *PloS One* 9, no. 5 (January 2014): e97927, doi:10.1371/journal.pone.0097927.

59. U.S. Department of Health and Human Services, "2008 Physical Activity Guidelines for Americans."

60. Ross C. Brownson, Tegan K. Boehmer, and Douglas A. Luke, "Declining Rates of Physical Activity in the United States: What Are the Contributors?," *Annual Review of Public Health* 26 (October 7, 2005): 421–43.

61. Ibid.

62. Ibid.

63. Uri Ladabaum et al., "Obesity, Abdominal Obesity, Physical Activity, and Caloric Intake in US Adults: 1988 to 2010," *American Journal of Medicine* 127, no. 8 (August 2014): 717–727.e12, doi:10.1016/j.amjmed.2014.02.026.

64. The Exercise Is Medicine campaign is dedicated to making exercise a standard part of disease prevention and to include questions about physical activity in all patient visits. It is endorsed by hundreds of health-related organizations. The list can be found at http://www.exerciseismedicine.org/supporters.htm.

65. Susan A Carlson et al., "Trend and Prevalence Estimates Based on the 2008 Physical Activity Guidelines for Americans," *American Journal of Preventive Medicine* 39, no. 4 (October 2010): 305–13, doi:10.1016/j.amepre.2010.06.006.

66. Jared M. Tucker, Gregory J. Welk, and Nicholas K. Beyler, "Physical Activity in U.S.: Adults Compliance with the Physical Activity Guidelines for Americans," *American Journal of Preventive Medicine* 40, no. 4 (April 2011): 454–61, doi:10.1016/j.amepre.2010.12.016.

67. Ibid.

68. Ibid. Accelerometers aren't perfect, and they are more likely to underestimate exercise than to overestimate it.

69. Ryan E. Rhodes and Gert-Jan de Bruijn, "How Big Is the Physical Activity Intention-Behaviour Gap? A Meta-Analysis Using the Action Control Framework," *British Journal of Health Psychology* 18, no. 2 (May 2013): 296–309, doi:10.1111/bjhp.12032.

70. Geoff Williams, "The Heavy Price of Losing Weight," *U.S. News & World Report*, January 2, 2013, http://money.usnews.com/money/personal-

finance/articles/2013/01/02/the-heavy-price-of-losing-weight.   Williams cites: "Gym Membership Statistics," StatisticsBrain.com, 2012, http://www.statisticbrain.com/gym-membership-statistics/.

71.   Thirty billion dollars per year are spent on fitness clothes in the United States, according to sportsbusinessdaily.com, cited in: Amber Goodfellow, "The Athletic Apparel Industry: Fitness or Fashion?," *Digital Universe*, 2013, http://universe.byu.edu/2013/07/30/the-athletic-apparel-industry-fitness-or-fashion/.

72.   Entire books and thousands of articles have been written on this point alone. This book is a nice summary: Mark Conner et al., *Predicting Health Behaviour* (Maidenhead, England: McGraw-Hill International, 2005). This article is also helpful: Ralf Schwarzer, "Modeling Health Behavior Change: How to Predict and Modify the Adoption and Maintenance of Health Behaviors," *Applied Psychology* 57, no. 1 (January 2008): 1–29, doi:10.1111/j.1464-0597.2007.00325.x.

73.   Conner et al., *Predicting Health Behaviour.*

74.   Marcel den Hoed et al., "Heritability of Objectively Assessed Daily Physical Activity and Sedentary Behavior," *American Journal of Clinical Nutrition* 98, no. 5 (November 18, 2013): 1317–25, doi:10.3945/ajcn.113.069849.

75.   Justin S. Rhodes, Theodore Garland, and Stephen C. Gammie, "Patterns of Brain Activity Associated with Variation in Voluntary Wheel-Running Behavior," *Behavioral Neuroscience* 117, no. 6 (December 1, 2003): 1243–56, doi:10.1037/0735-7044.117.6.1243.

76.   Ibid.

77.   Rachel J. Burns et al., "A Theoretically Grounded Systematic Review of Material Incentives for Weight Loss: Implications for Interventions," *Annals of Behavioral Medicine* 44, no. 3 (December 2012): 375–88, doi:10.1007/s12160-012-9403-4.

78.   The student was Rachel Burns.

79.   Rachel J. Burns, "Can We Pay People to Act Healthily? Testing the Relative Effectiveness of Incentive Dimensions and Underlying Psychological Mediators," (University of Minnesota, 2014).

80.   I'm not alone in this experience. Benjamin Lorr describes something similar in his book (though he takes things a bit far). Benjamin Lorr, *Hell-Bent: Obsession, Pain, and the Search for Something Like Transcendence in Competitive Yoga* (New York: St. Martin's Press, 2012).

81.   The following makes the point that reinforcers need to be immediate: C. B. Ferster and B. F. Skinner, *Schedules of Reinforcement* (East Norwalk, CT: Appleton-Century-Crofts, 1957). I have not seen specific research evidence for the effectiveness of fitness feedback over weight feedback on long-term exercise maintenance. I am conducting research on this now.

82.   Carolina O. C. Werle, Brian Wansink, and Collin R. Payne, "Is It Fun or Exercise? The Framing of Physical Activity Biases Subsequent Snacking," *Marketing Letters* (May 15, 2014), doi:10.1007/s11002-014-9301-6.

83.   Staub, "Instigation to Goodness"; Howland, Hunger, and Mann, "Friends

Don't Let Friends Eat Cookies."

84.   Staub, "Instigation to Goodness"; Howland, Hunger, and Mann, "Friends Don't Let Friends Eat Cookies."

85.   Gollwitzer and Sheeran, "Implementation Intentions and Goal Achievement."

86.   Sarah Milne, Sheina Orbell, and Paschal Sheeran, "Combining Motivational and Volitional Interventions to Promote Exercise Participation: Protection Motivation Theory and Implementation Intentions," *British Journal of Health Psychology* 7, no. Pt 2 (May 2002): 163–84, doi:10.1348/135910702169420.

87.   Ibid.

88.   Gollwitzer and Sheeran, "Implementation Intentions and Goal Achievement."

89.   Williams, "The Heavy Price of Losing Weight."

90.   Schwartz et al., "Healthier by Precommitment."

91.   E. Kahn et al., "The Effectiveness of Interventions to Increase Physical Activity: A Systematic Review," *American Journal of Preventive Medicine* 22, no. 4 (May 2002): 73–107, doi:10.1016/S0749-3797(02)00434-8; G. Neil Thomas et al., "Health Promotion in Older Chinese: A 12-Month Cluster Randomized Controlled Trial of Pedometry and 'Peer Support,'" *Medicine and Science in Sports and Exercise* 44, no. 6 (June 2012): 1157–66, doi:10.1249/MSS.0b013e318244314a.

FINAL WORDS: DIET SCHMIET

1.   Tomiyama et al., "Low Calorie Dieting Increases Cortisol."

2.   Glennon Doyle Melton, "Your Body Is Not Your Masterpiece," Momastery blog, July 6, 2014, http://momastery.com/blog/2014/07/06/body-masterpiece/.

INDEX

Page numbers of illustrations appear in italics.
The letter "n" refers to endnotes.

ABOUT THE AUTHOR

Traci Mann is professor of social and health psychology at the University of Minnesota. She received her Ph.D. in psychology from Stanford University and was a tenured professor at UCLA before moving to the University of Minnesota in 2007, where she founded the Health and Eating Lab. Her research has been funded by the National Institutes of Health, the United States Department of Agriculture, and the National Aeronautics and Space Association (NASA). She lives with her husband, University of Minnesota professor of psychology Stephen Engel, and their two sons in Edina, Minnesota.